OUTLIVE WORKBOOK

*The Ultimate Interactive Guide to Unlock Attia's Insights | Includes Practical
Exercises, Reflection Questions, Key Points & Much More*

AMBROSE SACKLER

TABLE OF CONTENTS

INTRODUCTION

Setting Your Longevity Goals

The longevity of the human species is something that has always been a highly desired goal. Since the dawn of human history, people have been obsessed with finding out how to live longer, whether it is via myths about fabled locations like the Fountain of Youth or through the rigorous scientific investigation that goes into anti-aging research today. But increasing the number of years we have left in our lives isn't the only goal of people who want longevity; it's also about improving the quality of those years. To put it simply, defining your longevity objectives involves striking a fundamental balance between the length of your life and its vibrancy.

To begin, it is necessary to specify what you understand by the term "longevity." Does it imply being able to participate in physical activities with your grandkids and maybe even your great-grandchildren, or does it mean surviving beyond the century mark without suffering from any kind of chronic illness? Perhaps it's the hope that you'll be able to keep your mind as clear and as sharp as possible far into your senior years. Understanding one's own perspective on what constitutes a long and healthy life is the first step in establishing goals that are both attainable and significant.

By incorporating healthy behaviors into your everyday routine, you are laying the basis for a long and healthy life. For example, proper nutrition is an essential component of this. The old saying "you are what you eat" is ringing truer than it ever has before as contemporary research continues to find the connections between nutrition and the consequences of one's health over the course of their lifetime. Consuming a diet that is well-rounded, high in antioxidants, lean proteins, and whole grains, as well as an abundance of fruits and vegetables, might help decrease the risk of developing chronic illnesses and may even slow down the aging process. It is important to keep in mind that the food we eat does more than simply provide energy for our bodies; it also nourishes the cells, tissues, and body part in our bodies, giving us the components necessary for a longer and better life.

Another essential component of a long and healthy life is regular exercise. It is generally established that engaging in regular physical activity may promote mental well-being, as well as the health of the cardiovascular system, bone density, and muscular tone. It's not only about the level of intensity; consistency is also important. Maintaining an active and supple body should be the focus of whatever physical practice you choose, be it brisk walking, yoga, or strength training. When it comes to our quality of life as we become older, it is not our chronological age that matters but rather our mobility, strength, and energy.

Both one's physical and mental health are essential components of a healthy and long life. Keeping our cognitive abilities intact, fostering healthy connections with others, and effectively managing stress all have a significant bearing on how long we live. Increasing mental resilience may be accomplished through engaging in cognitively challenging activities, practicing mindfulness, maintaining social connections, and ensuring enough sleep. The brain, just like any other muscle in the body, requires regular training, which should involve the taking on of new tasks, the acquisition of new knowledge, and the development of new experiences.

When you set your sights on living a long life, you should also familiarize yourself with and welcome advances in medical knowledge. At this point in time, we are living in a golden age of biotechnological innovation, during which researchers are exploring potential treatments at the cellular and even genetic levels. We can be at the vanguard of customized and preventive medicine if we take an active role in our health screenings, remain current on the most recent medical discoveries, and have open lines of communication with medical specialists.

In addition, it is of the utmost importance to be conscious of the fact that living a long life is not only a matter of one's own personal journey; rather, it is intricately connected to our surroundings. In our pursuit of longer, more meaningful lives, the environments in which we live, the quality of the air we take in, and the relationships we cultivate within our communities all play critical roles. The extent to which we live in healthy settings, limit our contact with harmful substances, and participate in communities that are supportive of one another may have a major impact on how long we live.

Objectives of the Workbook

Demystify Longevity Science: This workbook aims to demystify the science of longevity by providing readers with a comprehensive grasp of the most recent scientific discoveries linked to the biology of aging, genetics, and the consequences of these topics on human life.

Practical Application of Knowledge: To transform complex scientific ideas into practicable tactics and habits that may be incorporated into one's daily life without disrupting their flow.

Holistic Well-Being: To place equal emphasis on one's physical health, emotional well-being, and nutritional intake in the context of living a long and healthy life. Encourage the adoption of an all-encompassing strategy for health care that takes into consideration the whole scope of the human experience.

Self-discovery and Assessment: By using quizzes and other forms of self-evaluation, you may help your readers obtain insights into their own personal health as well as their habits and predispositions, which will assist in the development of a tailored strategy for increasing lifespan.

Empowerment via Information: Provide the readers with the resources and the background information they need to make educated choices about their health, lifestyle, and overall well-being.

Strategies for Longevity: Lifelong learning should be encouraged by fostering a continuing sense of curiosity and a dedication to keeping up with the most recent research and results in the area of longevity.

Customized Approaches to Longevity: By gaining an awareness of each reader's unique requirements and circumstances via the exercises in the workbook, you may assist readers in developing tailored approaches that will help them live longer and healthier lives.

Encourage Proactivity: Instill in people a mentality that sees longevity not as a result that is solely determined by heredity but rather as a result that conscious choices and behaviors can actively impact. This will encourage a more proactive approach to living a long and healthy life.

Stress the Importance of Mental Well-Being: Bring attention to the relevance of mental health, its relationship to physical health, and its role in the process of obtaining a longer life that is more meaningful.

How to Use this Workbook

Follow the instructions and guidelines below to get the most out of this workbook:

Open Your Mind

Some material may question your pre-existing assumptions about aging and health. Approach each segment with a sense of wonder and a readiness to learn.

Progress at Your Own Pace

Every trip is different. Some portions may need extra time for contemplation and comprehension. There's no need to hurry; take your time digesting the material.

Participate Actively

This workbook is intended to be interactive. Take the tests, perform the self-assessments, and immerse yourself in the activities. The more you invest, the more you will get.

Document Your Insights

Fill in the blanks with your ideas, insights, and findings. These notes will be useful references as you develop your unique longevity strategy.

Return Frequently

Longevity is a never-ending quest. Your demands and comprehension will change as you get older. Revisit areas on a regular basis to refresh your memory or adjust to new discoveries.

Apply What You Learn

Knowledge is most effective when it is put to use. Incorporate the methods and suggestions into your everyday life. Experiment, tweak, and discover what works best for you.

Keep Up to Date

The subject of longevity research is always expanding. While this workbook offers a solid basis, consider searching out other materials, the most recent research, or expert viewpoints to keep current.

Build a Support System

Share your findings with your friends and family. Encourage conversation, form accountability groups, and even hold short seminars. A trip taken together might be more gratifying and encouraging.

Seek Professional Help

While this workbook provides broad information, everyone's requirements are unique. Consult appropriate specialists or experts for individualized advice, particularly on health or nutrition.

Celebrate Small Victories

While longevity is a long-term objective, every step matters. Celebrate the good changes, new habits, and accomplishments. This will keep you going.

Part 1:
THE SCIENCE OF LONGEVITY

Chapter 1:
Understanding the Biology of Aging

The aging process is something that all of us are familiar with, along with its telltale indications, which include aching joints, graying hair, and wrinkles that demonstrate how much we've laughed over the years. But most of us don't have a good grasp on what is taking on in our bodies as we get older or what this implies for the myriad components of our bodies and how they operate.

Our Body's Organs and Cells

Each day, some of the cells in our body will die and be replaced by brand-new cells that have just been created. When we age, some of our cells pass away naturally, sometimes due to being designed to do so and sometimes because of being harmed.

The death of these cells has an effect on our organs and the operation of those organs. Because older cells do not operate as well, our organs, including our heart, kidneys, lungs, and brain, begin to work less effectively as we age. This decline in function may be traced back to the aging of our cells. When our bodies are in better shape, more of the cells in our organs can carry out their functions.

Our Skeleton and its Muscles

Many of us become shorter as we get older, often losing approximately two inches in height by the time we reach the age of 80. This is due, in large part, to the vertebrae in our spine becoming compressed, as well as, in part, to alterations in our legs and feet.

We also discover that as we get older, a greater proportion of our muscle mass is converted into fat, increasing by an average of 14–30% between the ages of 25 and 75. If you consider that this has a lot to do with the makeup of hormones in our bodies as an excuse to slack off when controlling your food and exercise, you may easily exceed these averages much more quickly.

Along with fat accumulation, our muscles will undergo attrition, reducing size and strength. In most cases, this is immediately followed by bone loss, which occurs when our bones slow down their healing processes, causing them to become thinner and more porous. This will also be accompanied by a reduction in the cartilage found in our joints (which is why, as we age, our joints get progressively uncomfortable because of the increased strain placed on them).

Our Nose and Mouth Together

When we reach our 50s, most of us won't even be aware of the slow decline in our sense of taste or smell that occurs throughout this time. As we age, the taste buds in our mouth become less sensitive, and we find that we can detect sweet and salty flavors better than bitter and sour ones. Our sense of smell also declines, which means that we can distinguish fewer of the subtleties present in complex flavors and cuisines.

The Human Brain

The number of nerve cells in an individual with a healthy brain will gradually but steadily decline with time. However, new connections are established to compensate for the loss of cells, new clusters are utilized, and redundant functional groups are created. As we age, the receptors in our skin that carry messages to the brain can deteriorate, implying that our perception of touch and pain would shift. This may result from a decrease in spinal fluid or any of a number of other potential causes.

Because of the increased risk of stroke, Alzheimer's disease, or dementia as we age, exercising our brains is just as vital as exercising the rest of our bodies.

Our Eyes

The majority of individuals are totally unaware of the fact that our eyes start the process of changing very early on in adulthood. Like most other organs, the eyes reach their maximum level of functionality around the age of 30, after which they begin a steady decline that continues into old life. Physically, the lenses of the eyes have a tendency to harden and get thicker, which makes it more difficult to see in low light circumstances or concentrate the way they used to be able to. The muscles that control the pupil's size respond to shifts in illumination more slowly, and the number and health of the eye's nerve cells deteriorate as the condition progresses. As people become older, their eyes also begin to generate less fluid, which can occasionally cause irritation and dryness in the eye.

Most people, in general, first become aware of these changes to their eyes when they experience a gradual decrease in the clarity of their vision throughout their lifetime. People frequently discover that they require more light than normal, have greater trouble differentiating colors, or struggle to see writing up close (which often leads them to reach for "readers").

Our Hair

Even though a wide variety of cosmetics are available to disguise gray hair, having gray hair has become a fashion statement. Even Glamour referred to this extraordinary era as the "gray-hair revolution." But here's a news flash: You don't have to wait for gray hair to become fashionable before you can flaunt it since it's entirely natural! Your hair will begin to gray naturally as you get older. Your hair color might shift due to your hair follicles producing less melanin (a pigment) as you age. This applies to all of the hair on your body, including the hair in your armpits and pubic area. It is common for this to start happening while you're in your 30s, but it can begin to happen much younger for certain people. Your hair will turn white at some point in the future.

Additionally, as you get older, the thickness of your hair will vary. This is because each strand of protein that makes up your hair is something your body generates less and less of as time goes on. The average lifespan of a single hair is between two and seven years, and the pace at which your hair grows naturally slows down as you get older, so it is natural for you to experience some thinning and even some balding as you get older. It is also possible that some follicles will cease generating hair completely.

Your senses

Your perceptions of smell and taste are susceptible to change as you age, whether for the better or the worse. As you age, you'll find that strong, unpleasant odors don't bother your nose as much, but you won't be able to smell the pleasant things quite as clearly.

It's interesting to note that your sense of smell plays a significant part in retrieving memories. It doesn't matter if you take a whiff of perfume or a flower; just the scent of something might bring up warm and fuzzy memories of reminiscence. But all of that might change as time goes on. The inability to smell can also significantly diminish the flavor of meals. When food does not have the same mouthwatering appeal as it once had, we tend to load it up with unhealthful additions such as, you know, salt and sugar.

The hazard posed by these chemicals increases with age, particularly if the individual develops a medical condition such as high blood pressure or blood sugar. To add insult to injury, the drugs used to treat these diseases might sometimes alter the meal's flavor. In addition, if you smoke cigarettes and don't practice good dental hygiene for your whole life, you could get a rancid taste in your mouth.

Self-Assessment Questions

1. "What are some common physical changes that occur as people age?"

   Answer

2. "Can you name three factors that contribute to the aging process?"

   Answer

3. "How does a healthy lifestyle influence the aging process?"

   Answer

4. "What are the primary challenges that elderly individuals may face?"

   Answer

5. "Do you know the difference between chronological age and biological age? Explain."

   Answer

6. "What is the significance of mental health in the context of aging?"

Answer

7. "List three ways in which technology has impacted the lives of seniors.

Answer

8. "How does social interaction affect the well-being of older adults?

Answer

9. "Name three common misconceptions about aging. Are they true or false?"

Answer

10. "Explain the concept of 'successful aging' and its key components."

Answer

Creating Your Biological Age Profile

These are the main things to be included when creating your profile:

1. **Age:** You must be aware of your true age. It's like the beginning point for this whole journey.

2. **Health Questionnaire**: A series of questions about your life, habits, and medical history will be required. Questions about your food, fitness regimen, smoking, and drinking habits.

3. **Physical Exam**: It's time for a check-up! Your blood pressure, fat levels, and body mass index (BMI) will all be measured. They may also check your heart rate and do a stethoscope dance on your chest.

4. **Blood Tests**: Blood tests play an important role in this profile. examine numerous blood indicators such as glucose, lipids, and inflammatory markers. It's like your blood giving you its tale.

5. **DNA Testing**: Some profiles go over and above by including DNA testing. Examine your DNA to determine if you have any hidden genetic characteristics that may be impacting your biological age.

6. **Lifestyle Factors**: Your biological age may be influenced by your sleeping habits, stress levels, and even the number of friends you have. It's like a puzzle, and every piece is important.

7. **Medical History:** It doesn't matter what medical ailments you've had, what operations you've had, or what drugs you're taking.

8. **Family History:** If some illnesses run in your family, your biological age may be affected as well.

9. **Nutritional Habits:** What you eat is important. Your food may have a significant impact on how your body matures.

CHAPTER 2:
GENETICS AND EPIGENETICS

There is a lot of controversy around the concept of longevity, and the fact that there isn't one widely accepted definition increases the likelihood of erroneous interpretations and biases when contrasting the results of various research that seek to determine the influence of genetics on this characteristic. In addition, the phrases lifetime, oldest old, aging, and longevity are often used interchangeably across academic research. Longevity may be described as the consequence of overall mortality selection age groups, where cumulative mortality is based on historical background and present-day circumstances. As a result, the chronological age itself is not the most important factor in the definition of longevity; rather, the birth cohort and the percentile of survival are two significant characteristics. There are disparities between individuals of a birth cohort who live 90, 100, 106, and 110+ years, as shown by demographic research; these discrepancies may thus indicate major genetic variances. The relative chance of siblings surviving to older ages increases with age. This discovery lends credence to the hypothesis that the amount of impact exerted by genetics on survival steadily rises to its maximum point near the extreme reaches of the human lifetime.

This finding suggests that the ability to discover genetic associations with lifespan is higher among individuals who live to be 100 years old (centenarians) compared to those who live to be 90 years old (nonagenarians) within the same group of individuals born in the same time period. Hence, a recent scholarly article suggests that the concept of longevity should be delineated based on percentile survival, which is established by comparing the lifespan of individuals within a specific group to that of a reference birth cohort. This observation highlights the significance of the environmental context in shaping the expression of this particular trait. The author of the paper recommends implementing this measure in order to mitigate potential inconsistencies in the definition. The threshold for surviving at the first percentile is identified as the lowest need for maximizing the probability of detecting genetic associations. In addition, the hereditary aspect of human longevity is a variable that is taken into account in studies pertaining to the genetic basis of lifespan. The Genetics of Healthy Aging Study (GEHA) incorporates sibling pairs in their selection process, specifically targeting nonagenarians, in order to identify families with a significant genetic influence on longevity.

Scientists and researchers have long been captivated by the genetics of longevity as they strive to untangle the complicated interaction between our genes, environmental variables, and the astonishing capacity of certain people to live far longer than the typical human lifetime. Significant discoveries have been made due to the search to understand why some individuals live to be 100 or older. These findings emphasize the complicated nature of human longevity.

The study of centenarians, or those who have accomplished the astounding milestone of living to 100 or more, is at the center of the genetics of longevity field. Centenarians are people who have lived their whole lives. Scientists have uncovered several genetic variations that are found in centenarians at a higher frequency than they are seen in the general population. This was accomplished via considerable study and genetic analysis. These genetic variants are often connected to biological processes, including the management of inflammation, the maintenance of cells, and the repair of DNA. The APOE gene is a well-known example since it has several variations, each linked with a varied risk for Alzheimer's and cardiovascular diseases. Certain APOE variations are found in centenarians, which are thought to contribute to the centenarians' longer lifespans and superior cognitive performance.

Studies based on genetics have also shed light on telomeres' role in the aging process. Telomeres are the defensive caps at the ends of chromosomes, and they naturally become shorter with each cell division. Telomeres are also known as telomeric endcaps. Eventually, dangerously short telomeres might lead to the senescence or death of the cell. However, some people have telomeres that are far longer than average for their age, which suggests that their cells are maintained more healthily and may be a factor in their longer lifespans. There is a correlation between variations in genes involved in the preservation of telomeres, such as the TERT and TERC genes, and longer telomeres, which have been related to enhanced lifespan.

The research on longevity genetics has shed light on the significance of gene-environment interactions and the individual genetic differences that have been uncovered. Our genetic makeup is not the only element that determines our lifespan; our longevity is affected by how our genes interact with the many aspects of our environment. The decisions we make about our food, our level of physical activity, and our group of exposure to stress are all important factors in deciding how our genes finally manifest themselves and how long we live. The effects of caloric restriction serve as a prime example of the interaction between genetics and the environment. It has been demonstrated that lowering calorie intake without leading to malnutrition can increase lifespan in various organisms. This could be the result of caloric restriction affecting genetic pathways related to metabolism and cellular stress resistance.

The study of epigenetics, which provides light on how gene expression may be affected by external stimuli, has been made possible by advancements in genomics technology, which have enabled epigenetics to be studied. DNA methylation and histone alterations are epigenetic changes that may impact gene function without changing the underlying genetic coding. According to the findings of many studies, some epigenetic patterns are linked to the aging process and disorders connected with aging. It has been shown that epigenetic alterations may play a significant role in maintaining cellular health and resilience. Centenarians generally display specific epigenetic profiles that contribute to their extraordinary lifespan.

The study of individual genes has given way to an investigation of the larger genomic landscape in longevity genetics, which has seen significant expansion in recent years. Genome-wide association studies, often known as GWAS, entail evaluating the genetic data of large populations to uncover genetic differences related to certain attributes, such as lifespan. The results of these investigations have encountered several genetic loci associated with an exceptionally long lifespan, therefore shedding light on various biological processes that contribute to longevity. Nevertheless, the aggregate impact of these genetic differences is often not very significant, highlighting the complex polygenic character of the human lifespan.

Epigenetic Markers

The study of heritable characteristics that are not directly linked to changes in DNA sequence is called epigenetics. DNA methylation, histone modification, and the act of noncoding RNA are the three categories of epigenetic regulation that are now known. Epigenetic regulation affects the progression of development, differentiation, and the expression or susceptibility to illness in the cardiovascular system. Determining the factors that influence epigenetic regulation opens the door to developing innovative approaches to treating and preventing infection.

The term "epigenetics" was first used to describe the intricate relationship between a person's DNA and the external variables that influence the differentiation and development of cells and organs. At the moment, this word refers to heritable characteristics that are not a result of changes that occur in the sequence of DNA. These characteristics are the end consequence of changes in gene expression that were controlled by variations in the accessibility of DNA or the structure of chromatin. DNA methylation, the post-translational modification of histone proteins, and the activities of noncoding RNA in the nucleus may all be responsible for epigenetic alterations, also known as tags, which can result in changes in the extent to which DNA is accessible. Exogenous stimuli and environmental exposures may have an effect on epigenetic alterations, which establishes a mechanical relationship between genes (also known as the genome) and the environment (also known as the exposome) in the process of defining phenotype and provides an explanation for phenotypic variances that can occur between monozygotic twins. The study of epigenetics is experiencing a period of tremendous expansion. The idea that epigenetic changes have a role in the development of cardiovascular disease and the manifestation of cardiovascular pathophenotypes is gaining more and more support as scientific research continues.

Types of Epigenetic Markers

Chromatin structure

Chromatin is composed of nuclear DNA that is intricately connected with certain proteins at the atomic level. The process of DNA coiling around histone proteins, resulting in the formation of nucleosomes, is a well-established phenomenon. Each nucleosome consists of a central core composed of eight histone proteins, specifically two H3-H4 histone dimers and two H2A-H2B dimers. These histone proteins are intricately associated with a 147-base-pair segment of DNA. The H1 histone protein exhibits an affinity for the internucleosomal DNA linker sequences. The determination of chromatin structure is contingent upon the spacing of nucleosomes and can be classified into two categories: transcriptionally inactive heterochromatin, characterized by tight packing, and transcriptionally permissive euchromatin, characterized by less dense packing. Biochemical alterations to DNA and the aminoterminal histone tails, which extend from the nucleosome into the nuclear lumen, play a crucial role in regulating the chromatin shape and its impact on gene expression.

Methylation of DNA

The primary epigenetic change of DNA is the covalent addition of a methyl group to the C5 site of cytosine. This alteration is more common in CpG dinucleotide-containing regions, often in regulatory sequences restricting gene expression. CpG methylation is required for transposon and repeat element transcriptional repression, imprinting and X-chromosome inactivation, and tissue-specific gene expression throughout development and differentiation. Methylation of cytosines not inside CpG sequences may also occur and is critical for gene expression control in embryonic stem cells.

The process of methylation of cytosine has been observed to have two separate impacts on the control of transcription. Firstly, it can repress transcription by hindering the binding of transcription factors. Secondly, it can boost the binding of other transcriptional repressors, such as histone-modifying proteins like histone deacetylases (HDACs). The enzymatic activity responsible for cytosine methylation at CpG dinucleotides is facilitated by a class of enzymes referred to as DNA methyltransferases (DNMTs). The enzyme family under consideration includes DNMT3a and DNMT3b, which are accountable for the process of de novo methylation. Additionally, DNMT1 plays a crucial role in recognizing and methylating the daughter strand that lacks methylation during the replication of DNA. The principles of base-pairing facilitate the preservation of reciprocal methylation during consecutive DNA replication cycles, so enabling the transmission of a non-genetic trait from one cell to another. DNA methylation is commonly regarded as a durable and permanent epigenetic attribute.

Although it is well-recognized that demethylation is an important process that occurs throughout certain phases of development, the mechanism of DNA demethylation is far less well-understood than the mechanism of methylation. Loss of methylation, either specifically targeted or globally, has been linked to various diseases, including cancer, cardiovascular disease, and others. Demethylation may be key in modulating brain plasticity or transcriptional responses to hormones. The inhibition of DNMT1 methyl transferase may lead to widespread reductions in the amount of methylation seen in DNA. According to recent studies, it has been discovered that demethylation can potentially take place via alternate enzymatic pathways, which rely on excision-repair mechanisms to substitute methylcytosine with cytosine subsequent to deamination. The presence of these processes is essential for the occurrence of demethylation. These processes have the potential to induce alterations in methylation patterns on a broad or specific level. The enzymatic activity of the ten-eleven translocation (Tet) enzymes is accountable for the process of oxidizing methyl cytosines, resulting in the formation of hydroxymethyl cytosine. This represents one of the potential mechanisms underlying the process of demethylation. There is an increasing body of information that suggests the involvement of hydroxymethyl cytosine as an intermediary component in the DNA demethylation process. One possible explanation for this phenomenon could be attributed to the heightened susceptibility of hydroxymethyl cytosine to deamination.

Nevertheless, the role of Tet proteins appears to be crucial in the process of replication-independent DNA demethylation. The potential existence of further crucial functions of five hydroxymethyl cytosine as an epigenetic marker, capable of regulating gene expression and chromatin structure, remains uncertain.

Histone alterations

Histones undergo many posttranslational modifications, such as acetylation, methylation, phosphorylation, and ubiquitination, resulting in variations to chromatin structure and gene expression. The concept of the "histone code" posits that different types and combinations of modifications have distinct effects on chromatin structure and the capability for transcription. The acetylation of lysine residues in the aminoterminal tails of histones H3 and H4, specifically targeting the -amino group, has been extensively investigated as a histone modification that enhances transcriptional activity in many instances. Histone acetyltransferases are responsible for the catalysis of histone acetylation. This process is assisted by transcriptional cofactors, including cyclic AMP response element-binding protein and p300. There is a correlation between CpG methylation and the adoption of an inactive chromatin conformation, which is associated with histone deacetylation. There are four distinct types of histone deacetylases (HDACs) that facilitate the process of deacetylation. These HDACs are subject to regulation by posttranslational modifications. Histone lysine methylation is a significant category of histone modifications that exert an influence on gene expression. Nevertheless, the factors that determine whether gene expression is repressed or promoted in relation to this modification are intricate. The comprehensive understanding of the specific role played by lysine residues and the extent of methylation in influencing these activities is still lacking. Histone methylation, akin to histone acetylation, exhibits a notable level of reversibility. This process encompasses the enzymatic activities of numerous histone lysine methyltransferases and demethylases, which exhibit selectivity towards particular lysine residues and govern the mono-, di-, or trimethylation statuses.

Noncoding RNA

Long noncoding RNAs have the ability to induce gene silencing by their interaction with remodeling complexes, such as the polycomb complex, which in turn promote histone methylation. This is one of the processes by which they attain this impact. Furthermore, these ribonucleic acids (RNAs) possess the ability to recruit RNA-binding proteins, so potentially restricting the binding of transcription factors to promoter regions or impeding the process of histone deacetylation. Long noncoding RNAs (lncRNAs) are essential for the processes of imprinting and X-chromosome inactivation. Additionally, they play significant roles in cardiac development. The functions of lncRNAs are mediated through these processes and others. Previous studies have demonstrated the involvement of short noncoding RNAs, small inhibitory RNAs, and dicer-dependent microRNAs in the process of transcriptional repression, employing diverse strategies. One of the mechanisms involved in this process entails the recruitment of specific argonaute proteins for the purpose of assembling epigenetic remodeling complexes. These complexes facilitate the process of histone deacetylation, histone methylation, and DNA methylation. World-interacting RNAs (wiRNAs) are a specific type of short noncoding RNAs that are characterized by their single-stranded nature. It has been empirically established that they play a crucial role in the preservation of RNA-induced epigenetic silencing that is passed down from one generation to the next. The length of these RNAs varies between 21 and 30 nucleotides.

The Epigenetics of RNA

RNA epigenetics is a kind of post-transcriptional epigenetics that refers to alterations made to RNA after transcription. For instance, RNA (including tRNA, mRNA, and rRNA) may undergo methylation at several places in the nucleotide base and at the two positions of the ribose, and these methylation events might affect function. Methylation can also occur at the three positions of the ribose. There are four families that make up the RNA methyltransferases, and S-adenosylmethionine is used by all of them as a universal methyl donor. In addition, there is evidence that RNA demethylases may be involved in regulating gene expression. The methylation of RNA may have various effects on its activity, including stability, enhancement of function, and regulation of quality. For instance, changes may contribute to the tertiary structure of tRNA as well as the precision with which tRNA is recognized. These alterations can be detected in certain areas of tRNA. RNA epigenetics is a relatively new area still in its early stages of development. Still, it can potentially add another layer of complexity to the epigenetic control of gene expression.

Quiz: Genetic Health Assessment

Family History:

a. Do you have a family history of certain genetic disorders or diseases? (For example, cancer, heart disease, or diabetes)

b. If so, please write the ailments you have and any pertinent facts.

Ancestry:

a. Do you know anything about your ancestors? (For example, European, Asian, African, and so on.)

b. Are there any recognized genetic disorders that run in your family tree?

Personal Health:

a. Have you ever had a hereditary ailment or disease diagnosed?

b. Have you had any health problems that have plagued you for the most of your life?

Lifestyle Factors:

a. Do you smoke or have a smoking history?

b. Do you have a history of substance abuse or alcoholism?

c. Do you eat a well-balanced diet and exercise on a regular basis?

Environmental Factors:

a. Have you been exposed to any harmful substances or risks that may have an impact on your health?

Family Planning:

a. Do you intend to have children or do you currently have them?

b. Have you thought about genetic counseling or testing for family planning?

CHAPTER 3:
NUTRITION FUNDAMENTALS

Macronutrients

Macronutrients maintain the structure and function of your body, the primary types of nutrients present in your diet. You normally need a substantial quantity of macronutrients to support your body functioning at its optimal level. But don't worry; your body gets the energy it needs from calories from the macronutrients it consumes, which come from proteins, lipids, and carbs.

Measuring macros in grams (g) is common practice, which may be an effective approach to keeping tabs on the food you consume.

One may want to count their macronutrients to ensure that they are meeting their needs and that they are not overconsuming or underconsuming particular nutrients.

Instead of focusing on the number of calories you consume, you may switch your attention to the type of meals you consume and the quantity of each by counting macros. Even more specialized diets, such as the ketogenic and paleo diets, adhere to the macronutrient theory.

The following are examples of macronutrients:

- During digestion, the parts of meals most likely to be classified as belonging to one of the three categories of macronutrients are broken down and put to use in various ways. These are examples of macronutrients:
- Composed of carbs. Carbohydrates are the primary energy source, and their breakdown into glucose facilitates digestion and a feeling of fullness. Bread, pasta, rice, cereals, fruits, and vegetables high in starch, beans, milk, and yogurt all contain carbohydrates. They have a calorie density of 4 per gram.
- Fat. When fats are digested, they are converted into fatty acids and glycerol, which in turn provide the body with fat-soluble vitamins A, D, E, and K. Nuts, seeds, oils, butter, sour cream, mayonnaise, and cream cheese are examples of foods that have nine calories for every gram.
- The protein. In addition to assisting in forming and repairing muscle, tissues, and organs, protein also plays a role in controlling hormones. Meat, chicken, fish, eggs, cheese, cottage cheese, plain Greek yogurt, and tofu provide four calories per gram.

Other foods that give as many calories per gram include cheese, cottage cheese, and tofu.

The following is a list of things that the Dietary Guidelines Include:

- Carbohydrate content ranges from 45–65 percent of total calories.
- 20–35 percent of total calories come from fat.
- 10–35 percent of total calories come from protein.

To count macros, you first need to calculate the average number of calories that you burn during the day. The next step is to determine how many calories, broken down into those three categories, you need to consume each day to achieve your objectives.

Everyone has their own unique set of priorities and objectives. One person may want to count macros to maintain a healthy weight, while another could be more interested in using them to help grow muscle or maintain blood sugar levels.

In addition, your percentages of different macronutrients may alter depending on factors such as your age, gender, certain medical problems, how you live your life, and the amount of physical activity you get.

However, counting macros requires a significant amount of arithmetic and might be challenging for most people to understand. In addition, no conclusive study supports the assertion that this strategy is successful. You may seek the assistance of a trained dietitian or a nutritionist to assist you in determining the diet that would work best for you.

Milligrams (mg), micrograms (mcg), and international units (IU) are the standard units of measurement for micronutrients, which include vitamins and minerals.

Your body requires a lower quantity of micronutrients to function at its best compared to the macronutrients it needs. Even though micronutrients do not generate energy, they are necessary for digestion, the generation of hormones, and proper brain function.

Although keeping tabs on your macronutrient intake might be useful, accurately measuring and estimating the amount of micronutrients you take in on a daily basis can be challenging.

These are some examples of micronutrients:

The foods you consume daily, such as fruits and vegetables, are good sources of micronutrients, just as they are of macronutrients.

"The majority of vitamins are water-soluble." This indicates that they are eliminated from your body via urination after your body has satisfied its need for those substances.

Examples of vitamins that also serve as examples of micronutrients include the following:

- Vitamin B1 (B1 Vitamin). Vitamin B1, often referred to as thiamine, is a nutrient that assists in transforming other nutrients into energy. A few examples of these foods include white rice, fortified morning cereals, and black beans.
- Vitamin B2 is referred to as B2. This vitamin is beneficial for the generation of energy, the operation of cells, and the metabolism of fat. It is also known as riboflavin. Foods that are included include fat-free yogurt, milk, and quick oats.
- Vitamin B3, also known as B3. Vitamin B3, often referred to as niacin, is an essential component in the process that converts food into usable energy. Foods consisting of breast meat include chicken, turkey, salmon, and tuna.
- Vitamin B5 is one example. This vitamin is also known as pantothenic acid, and it plays an important role in the production of fatty acids. Shiitake mushrooms, sunflower seeds, and avocados are all examples of foods.
- This is vitamin B6. Vitamin B6, also recognized as pyridoxine, is necessary for the production of red blood cells and assists in the release of sugar from carbs that have been stored in the body for use as energy. Foods such as chickpeas, tuna, and potatoes are included.
- Supplemental vitamin B7. It is also known as biotin and plays an significant role in the metabolism of glucose, amino acids, and fatty acids. Some examples of these foods include eggs, salmon, pork chops, and sweet potatoes.
- Vitamin B9; see also vitamin B7. Also known by the name folate. The correct division of cells requires a sufficient amount of vitamin B9. Foods such as spinach, fortified breakfast cereals, white rice, and asparagus are rich in iron.
- Vitamin B12 is also known as cobalamin. Vitamin B12, also recognized by its chemical name cobalamin, contributes to the development of healthy red blood cells and to normal brain and nervous system function. Foods such as cow liver, salmon, milk, and yogurt are examples.

The nutrient vitamin C. Vitamin C, also known as ascorbic acid, is necessary for the production of neurotransmitters and collagen. Foods containing red peppers, oranges, grapefruits, and kiwis are included.

The following are some examples of minerals that are considered micronutrients:

- The mineral calcium. This inorganic is important for the proper function of bones, teeth, and muscles, and it also helps produce strong bones and teeth. Some examples of foods include cheese, milk, yogurt, and orange juice.
- The mineral magnesium. This mineral, which may be found in foods such as pumpkin seeds, almonds, and spinach, controls blood pressure.

- Salt is made of sodium. You need salt to keep your blood pressure at a healthy level and achieve the appropriate fluid balance in your body.
- Electrolyte that is potassium. Potassium is important for the proper functioning of muscles and nerve transmission. Potassium is found in various foods, including apricots, lentils, prunes, and raisins.

The Role of Diet in Longevity

To live a long life is the goal of the pursuit of longevity. We could want to live a long life to spend many years spending quality time with our loved ones or have the opportunity to see the globe. But if old age brings with it the burdens of illness or infirmity, it does not always guarantee that one will be healthy or happy during their whole life span. Even though individuals live more years in poor health, the population of people over 65 has expanded more swiftly than the number of people in other age groups owing to higher life spans and lower birth rates. For this reason, we won't simply focus on a person's lifetime but also their health span, which aims to maximize the years spent in good health.

The axis of sugar and the endocrine system

On the other hand, sugars have been proven to play a significant part in the signaling process, speeding up the aging process. The researchers found that mice with their adenylyl cyclase (AC) type 5 disrupted had a 30% longer median life span and a reduced incidence of cardiomyopathy than mice that did not have their AC type 5 disrupted. AC type 5 is largely found in the brain and the heart. Additionally, the disruption of the protein kinase A (PKA) RIIb subunit in male mice was related to increased lifespan, lower glucose and insulin levels when fasting, and a decreased incidence of left ventricular hypertrophy.

Fasting

The practice of intermittent fasting may achieve a longer lifespan. Fasting has several beneficial effects on the body, including better management of blood glucose, increased resilience to stress, less inflammation, and reduced formation of potentially dangerous free radicals. While cells are starved, broken molecules are either removed or repaired. The growth of chronic diseases, counting obesity, diabetes, cardiovascular disease, cancer, and neurological decline like Alzheimer's, may be avoided due to these impacts. In addition to these effects, animals who participate in intermittent fasting see improvements in their balance, coordination, and cognition, particularly in memory. In trials conducted on humans, researchers discovered that insulin sensitivity was enhanced, blood pressure was lowered, LDL cholesterol was reduced, and participants lost weight. However, further research on humans, including randomized controlled trials, is still required to fully understand the effects of fasting on aging and lifespan.

Here are five things you can do to live a longer and healthier life.

- **A healthy diet** - The incidence of hypertension, often known as high blood pressure, and dementia are known to rise with advancing age. Dietary patterns similar to those seen in the DASH, MIND, and Mediterranean diets, among others, have been shown to reduce the risk of developing chronic illnesses associated with advancing age. According to several large randomized controlled studies, taking a multivitamin and mineral supplement may also be of assistance in enhancing cognitive function and memory in some individuals.

- **Consistent physical activity** – The risk of various long-lasting infections, such as heart disease, high blood pressure, diabetes, osteoporosis, some malignancies, and cognitive decline, is reduced by engaging in regular physical exercise. A better quality of sleep, less worry, and lower blood pressure are all benefits of regular exercise. The first recommendation in the Physical Exercise Guidelines is to move more and sit less, with any training preferable to none. They recommend a minimum of 150–300 minutes per week of moderate to strenuous activity, such as brisk walking or rapid dancing, in addition to two days per week of muscle-strengthening activities to reap the added health advantages of this recommendation. Exercises focusing on maintaining balance, such as tai chi and yoga, might benefit seniors at risk of falling. Please see this page for other issues about older individuals' physical exercise.

- Weight that is considered to be within a healthy range is something that must be determined on an individual basis. Reviewing current health issues, the medical history of one's family, one's weight history, and the body type that is genetically inherited are all important factors to consider. Monitoring an increase in detrimental visceral "belly fat" and weight change from age 20 may be advantageous rather than relying on scale weight as a health measure.

- **Giving up smoking** - Because it encourages chronic inflammation and oxidative stress (a condition that may harm cells and tissues), smoking is a significant risk factor for several illnesses and conditions, including cancer, diabetes, cardiovascular disease, lung disorders, and early death. Smoking is detrimental to almost all of the body's organs. Giving up smoking knowingly lowers the likelihood of developing any of these illnesses linked to smoking.

- **Alcohol consumption in moderation** - According to the findings of recent studies, moderate alcohol use, which is defined as one drink per day for women and two drinks per day for men, is related to a decreased risk of developing type 2 diabetes, having a heart attack, and dying prematurely from cardiovascular disease. Consuming alcohol in low to moderate quantities may boost "good" cholesterol levels, also known as high-density lipoprotein (HDL), and avoid tiny blood clots that might clog arteries. However, alcohol use, particularly heavy drinking, is also related to risks of addiction, liver disease, and numerous forms of cancer. Because of this, it is a complicated subject that is best explored with your physician to assess your unique risk vs. benefit concerning alcohol consumption.

Food Diary: Tracking Your Nutritional Intake

Fundamental Data:

What gender are you?

a. How much weight do you now weigh (in kilos or pounds)?
b. How tall are you (in millimeters or feet/inches)?
c. Do you have any dietary restrictions or medical problems that influence your nutrition?

Dietary Objectives:

a. What are your key dietary objectives (for example, weight loss, muscle growth, increased energy levels, etc.)?
b. Are there any items you want to include or exclude from your diet?

Daily Food Journal:

a. Keep track of everything you eat and drink during the day.
b. Include serving amounts and cooking techniques (for example, grilled, steaming, or fried).
c. Take note of when each item was consumed.

Caloric Consumption:

a. How many calories do you intend to consume every day?
b. Have you assessed your Basal Metabolic Rate (BMR) or talked to a nutritionist about your calorie requirements?

Macronutrient Composition:

a. How much of your daily calorie intake should be made up of carbs, proteins, and fats?
b. Keep track of how many grams of each macronutrient you consume each day.
c. Consumption of fruits and vegetables:
d. How many portions of fruits and vegetables do you plan to consume each day?
e. Keep track of the types and amounts of fruits and vegetables you consume.

Sources of protein:

a. What are your primary protein sources (meat, fish, poultry, plant-based sources)?
b. How many grams of protein do you want to consume every day?

Hydration:

a. How much water or other beverages do you drink on a daily basis?
b. Do you have any specific hydration objectives in mind?

Snacking Patterns:

    a.   Do you like to nibble in between meals?

    b.   What kinds of snacks do you usually eat?

CHAPTER 4:
EXERCISE FOR LIFE

Movement performed purposefully, within a predetermined framework, and regularly is considered exercise. The four primary practice categories are Aerobic, strength, flexibility, and stability training. A steady workout has a wide range of positive effects on one's health, including enhancements to one's mental, cardiovascular, and structural well-being. In adding, investigation has shown that regular physical activity protects against various chronic illnesses, excessive weight gain, and obesity. It is generally agreed that maintaining a normal exercise routine is one of the most real ways to enhance one's health and extend one's life.

Types of Exercise and Their Benefits

1. Exercises that include aerobic movement

Aerobic activity is described as "requiring oxygen" in the dictionary. When you are involved in aerobic workout, the oxygen that you breathe in is transported to your muscles, where it is converted into the fuel that your body needs to function properly. Aerobic exercise is any physical activity that can be maintained for a prolonged time and involves big muscle groups. It is also often referred to as cardio exercise. Aerobic exercise may take many forms, including but not limited to walking, cycling, dancing, hiking, swimming, and running at a moderate speed.

2. Resistance training

Anaerobic exercise is a physical activity that includes the break of glucose (sugar) for energy without needing oxygen. Resistance training, also widely referred to as strength or weight training, is one form of anaerobic exercise. Utilizing one's body weight or an external resistance source, such as free weights or weight machines, the goal of strength training is to construct and keep one's muscular tissue in good condition. Workouts with weights are a great way to get key athletic groups, such as the legs, back, glutes, chest, shoulders, arms, and abdomen, stronger.

3. Flexibility

The range of motion that your joints are capable of and the mobility of your muscles are both components of flexibility. It is vital for sports performance and everyday functioning abilities and avoiding injuries if one has an acceptable amount of flexibility.

Static widening and dynamic widening are the two forms of stretching that are practiced the most often. Holding a stretch for a certain muscle group for a predetermined amount of time is what's meant by the term "static stretching." On the other hand, dynamic stretching is distinguished by active stretches that, most of the time, resemble a workout that will be done. Active and passive stretching are equally beneficial in enhancing flexibility and athletic performance. Static stretching is normally done after a workout when muscles are already more supple, but dynamic stretching is typically done before participating in physical activity to warm up muscles better. Dynamic stretching is generally suggested before physical exercise to warm up muscles.

4. Stability

Stability and balance exercises often include slow, controlled movements that activate and develop the core muscles, which are the muscles in your belly, back, and pelvis. These exercises may help improve your core strength and stability. All age groups may benefit from using these muscle groups via stability exercises, increasing a person's ability to perform day-to-day tasks such as ascending stairs, carrying heavy things, or rising from a chair. This kind of physical fitness is also called functional fitness in certain circles.

Instability, poor posture, and reduced athletic performance may all be caused by core muscles that are not strong enough. Include exercises that consistently activate numerous muscle groups in your program to enhance your stability and build stronger core muscles. Pushups, planks, and glute bridges are some examples of such exercises. In addition to being a well-liked type of exercise, Pilates is particularly effective in enhancing stability and core strength. Improving your balance and stability may also be accomplished by engaging in activities challenging your equilibrium, such as walking backward or standing on one leg at a time.

Health Benefits of Exercise

1. Promotes better cardiovascular and metabolic health

Because it can lower visceral fat, which is a form of fat deposited in the belly near essential organs, regular resistance exercise may be beneficial in avoiding and treating type 2 diabetes. A reduced amount of visceral fat not only increases insulin sensitivity but also brings down HbA1c, which is a measure of how well blood sugar is managed.

Aerobic exercise can promote cardiovascular health by facilitating oxygen supply to all body parts, lowering inflammatory stages, and increasing the size of blood vessels. In addition to dropping blood pressure, exercise has been shown to lower levels of low-density lipoproteins (LDL) cholesterol and triglycerides. All three of these parameters are contributors to the development of cardiovascular disease.

2. Protects the health of the bones and joints

The maintenance of current bone mass and the stimulation of new bone development are both achieved by weight training and aerobic activity. It has also been shown that elderly persons may maintain or enhance their bone mineral density by engaging in weight-bearing activity. In addition, research suggests that persons with osteoarthritis and other joint disorders may benefit from regular exercise because it reduces joint pain and improves joint function.

Getting young children who still have growing bones to do exercises that require them to bear weight is particularly crucial. The term "bone-strengthening exercises" may refer to various activities, including aerobic and muscle strength training. These include running, jumping rope, playing tennis, and hopscotch since they all result in a force being applied to the bones when the body hits the ground. This force contributes to the development of both muscle and bone.

The assumption that strength training poses a risk to a child's physical growth and mental development has been debunked by several recent research. Strength exercise is safe for children and adolescents after gaining the abilities necessary for balance and postural control, which normally happens around the age of eight in most cases. It is suggested that children and teenagers learn adequate safety, restrict resistance, and avoid powerlifting and bodybuilding until they have attained physical maturity. This is because these activities may be dangerous.

3. Raise both the amount of muscle and the level of strength

The gradual loss of power mass that begins in maturity continues throughout life. This condition is referred to as sarcopenia. Adults who lead a sedentary lifestyle have a significantly increased chance of experiencing rapid muscle mass loss, ranging from three to eight percent every decade.

It is never too late to begin an exercise routine to maintain or grow the muscle mass you already have. This is the good news. At any age, resistance training is an excellent method for building lean muscle mass and increasing strength. Resistance training increases muscle strength, gait speed, and overall physical performance in older persons, and There is a correlation between increased muscle mass and greater life expectancy. According to one research, persons with a greater muscle mass were more likely to survive longer than those with a lower muscle mass.

4. Could elevate one's mood

Keeping up with a regular workout regimen may have a promising impact on your mental health that lasts for a long time. According to one research, participants who participated in aerobic exercise for at least 10 to 30 minutes three times per week had fewer symptoms of anxiety and depression. Some examples of aerobic exercise are cycling and jogging. Children and adults alike may benefit from increased self-esteem and confidence thanks to regular exercise. In addition, research suggests that regular exercise might boost emotional resilience and enhance how one reacts to stress.

5. Assists in the maintenance of a fit weight

Calories may be burned by participating in any physical exercise. Consequently, a typical method for weight reduction and controlling one's weight is participation in physical activity. Physical exercise helps individuals maintain their weight, which may minimize the danger of excessive weight gain and obesity, according to a substantial body of data from the scientific community.

A group of 82 men and women participated in a randomized control experiment that evaluated the effects of walking in conjunction with a calorie-restricted diet to the results of a calorie-restricted diet alone. The group who followed a calorie-restricted diet and engaged in a walking routine for 12 weeks lost much more weight than those who only followed the diet.

Your metabolism, or the rate at which your body burns calories, will speed up due to your efforts to build muscle via exercise. In addition, severe aerobic exercise may increase the energy expended for many hours after the workout. Compared to the rate of energy expenditure after a day of rest, the rate of energy expenditure following a period of vigorous cycling that lasted 47 minutes and was performed at a high intensity resulted in an increase that lasted for 14 hours after the activity. It has been shown that high-intensity interval exercise (HIIT), which contains of short bursts of intense exercise followed by brief rest intervals, causes a rise in metabolic rate that lasts for many hours after the workout.

6. Increases both mobility and equilibrium.

Training the stability muscles strengthens the neuromuscular control system, a network of neurons and muscles answerable for movement and posture. As a result, balance is improved. Regular stability exercises may also help avoid injuries, especially those affecting the knees and ankles. Better mobility and flexibility are two benefits that may be gained through stretching before and after physical exercise.

Exercise Plan

There are a lot of fitness and diet programs out there, and many of them guarantee that anybody who follows them will see amazing results. However, these plans often fall short of their high promises. There is no such thing as an effective diet plan that is generic enough to apply to everyone. An extremely successful strategy for one individual may become a complete failure for another. Because of this, it is essential to have a tailored system that considers your specific circumstances — a personalized workout and diet routine developed with your particular objectives and fitness level in mind to achieve effective outcomes.

Strength Training

The primary muscles of your body, including those in your arms, legs, core, and back, will get a workout from these exercises. The final objective is to achieve maximum muscular mass. Because of this, your metabolism will speed up, making it simpler for you to shed pounds even while you are not actively engaging in physical activity. In addition, strength training helps tone your body, which enables you to create a fitter image even if the scale doesn't reflect it.

The following are some examples of exercises that are considered strength training:

- Use free weights such as kettlebells and dumbbells for resistance. These may be used for lifting, as in bicep curls, or added to conventional bodyweight workouts like squats or lunges to increase the difficulty of the movement.
- Using stationary exercise equipment to do weightlifting. A large number of individuals highly value home gyms due to their convenience.
- Exercises using just one's body weight and including resistance training. Exercises like planks, push-ups, leg lifts, and wall sits are excellent.
- Yoga. Certain yoga poses, like the warrior, may improve strength, flexibility, and mental clarity.

Flexibility

It is time to rethink your workout strategy, particularly if you have previously neglected to stretch before beginning your workout. Stretching exercises are essential for enhancing your posture and balance because of their positive effects on your muscles. They not only assist you in avoiding injuries but also aid in your recovery from existing ones. Being flexible enables you to participate in activities more easily and with reduced levels of discomfort.

To make your long-term objectives more feasible and feel more comfortable in the interim, a greater range of motion may go a long way. If you would want to increase your flexibility, you could attempt the following exercises and activities:

- Pilates
- Yoga.
- Tai chi
- Dance

Cardio

No matter how much you dislike it, cardiovascular exercise is essential to maintaining your health. Exercising consistently may help you reduce your chance of developing heart disease by elevating your heart rate.

One of the most important advantages of cardiovascular exercise is its flexibility. You may get your heart rate up via a wide variety of activities, and if you keep looking, you'll eventually discover at least one of them that you like doing or that is simple to maintain for an extended period. Some examples are as follows:

- Running
- Biking
- Cross-country skiing
- Brisk walks
- Machines such as the treadmill or elliptical
- Collection sports such as basketball, football, or volleyball
- Swimming
- Rowing
- Boxing
- HIIT workouts

It is not always easy to decide where to begin when so many wonderful choices are available. When in doubt, choose activities you can participate in often and do not need a significant investment of time or money.

Find enjoyable methods to include activity into your routine and look for inventive ways. For instance, if you walk briskly while walking the dog, you may consider it part of your daily cardiovascular workout. If you like viewing sports on TV, you can work out by riding a recumbent bike while watching the big game.

Create A Schedule

Even if you are equipped with SMART objectives, enjoyable hobbies, and the greatest of intentions, you may still find it difficult to schedule time for daily exercises. It's possible that your hectic schedule is to blame for some of these roadblocks. When your workout isn't expressly put on the program, it's easy to fall into the trap of vegging out on the sofa instead of getting your sweat on, especially if you tend to procrastinate.

Your frame of mind may be changed by building a good habit and letting go of the inner "should I or shouldn't I" disputes holding you back when you create a straightforward training program.

Write precisely which workouts you want to accomplish on which days and when. You can keep track of this information using a calendar or planner. Even better, put a reminder in your calendar on your phone. You'll be surprised by how gratifying something as simple as giving yourself a checkmark after a great exercise may feel.

Choose Your Nutrition Plan

Whether you agree or not, the adage that six-pack abs are created in the kitchen is somewhat accurate. If the majority of your diet consists of prepackaged meals that are high in simple carbohydrates as well as trans or saturated fats in excessive amounts, you may spend hours on the treadmill and still end up gaining weight.

Several healthful food regimens may complement your efforts in the gym. The "clean eating" and the "Mediterranean diet" are two common diets. Regardless of the path that most appeals to you, you should give extra consideration to plant-based diets. The eating of fresh fruits and vegetables and grains in their entire form is required daily. Aim for a well-balanced combination of protein, unsaturated fats, and carbs. Timing is another factor that may be considered; although some individuals swear by intermittent fasting, others merely try to restrict the amount of food they eat after midnight.

Develop A Routine For Your Meals

One of the most important aspects of eating healthfully is planning meals. If you plan and make healthful meals and snacks, you'll be less likely to give in to the temptation of packaged foods and drive-through restaurants. The time you save by preparing meals at home may be better used by increasing your physical activity.

To get started, you should look for dishes that are suitable for the diet that you have chosen. Create a shopping list and a few meal plans based on the recipes that seem appealing to you. You should only purchase the items on this list when you are in the shop.

Exercise Log: Track Your Physical Activity

Question

1. What is your main reason for keeping track of your physical activity?

Answer

2. How many days a week do you intend to be physically active?

Answer

3. What kinds of physical activities do you prefer?

Answer

4. Do you currently follow an exercise regimen or routine?

Answer

5. When is the best time for you to exercise?

Answer

6. How long do you usually devote to each fitness session?

Answer

7. Do you prefer physical exercises that take place inside or outside?

Answer

8. What fitness equipment or gear do you use?

Answer

9. Are you keeping track of your daily steps or distance walked?

Answer

10. Do you keep an eye on your heart rate when exercising? If so, how so?

Answer

11. Have you established any fitness objectives (for example, weight loss, muscle gain, or greater endurance)?

Answer

12. Are you maintaining a record of your workouts, including the date, time, and activity?

Answer

CHAPTER 5:
ADVANCED MEDICAL METRICS

Biomarkers

The term "biological markers" is sometimes abbreviated to "biomarkers," which refers to biological measurements of a condition. According to one definition, a biomarker is "a characteristic that is precisely measured and evaluated as an indicator of usual biological processes, pathogenic processes, or pharmacological responses to a therapeutic intervention."

Biomarkers are the measurements used for clinical evaluation, such as blood pressure or cholesterol level. They are used to monitor and forecast health conditions in individuals or across groups so that appropriate treatment interventions may be planned. Examples of biomarkers are blood pressure and cholesterol levels.

One may employ biomarkers alone or with other indicators when determining an individual's health or illness status.

There is a diverse selection of biomarkers in use today. Each biological system, such as the cardiovascular, metabolic, or immunological systems, has its unique set of biomarkers characteristic of that system. Many of these biomarkers may be measured moderately and are now included in standard medical checkups.

Checking your heart rate, blood pressure, cholesterol, triglyceride levels, and fasting glucose levels can be included in a general wellness check. When diagnosing illnesses like obesity and metabolic disorders, it is common practice to utilize body measures, including weight, body mass index (BMI), and waist-to-hip ratio.

Biomarkers are helpful in the diagnosis and prognosis of major conditions, including diabetes and cardiovascular disease. The attendance or absence of a disease or health condition may be deduced from the presence or absence of certain biomarkers, which, when taken together, can provide a comprehensive picture of an individual's state of health and suggest whether or not a diagnosis has to be made.

Types of Biomarker

1. Risk Biomarkers

The first group consists of biomarkers that indicate susceptibility or risk. These biomarkers can determine the chance that a person will acquire a certain illness or medical condition in the foreseeable future. For instance, a genetic test determining a tendency to breast cancer may be regarded as a susceptibility or risk biomarker for the disease. There is a correlation between mutations in some genes, such as the BRCA1 and BRCA2, and an increased likelihood of getting breast and ovarian cancer. Individuals who might benefit from greater monitoring, risk-reducing operations, or targeted medicines can be identified by testing for certain variants and identified through this process.

2. Diagnostic Biomarkers

The second category encompasses diagnostic biomarkers, which serve the purpose of identifying or confirming the presence of a disease or other medical condition. Diagnostic biomarkers can additionally furnish insights into the manifestations and indications of a pathological condition. Several instances of disease biomarkers include the subsequent examples:

The acronym PSA denotes prostate-specific antigen, a biomarker employed in the diagnostic and surveillance procedures for prostate cancer. The monitoring of disease progression or response to treatment can be facilitated by tracking the fluctuations in PSA levels over a period of time. High levels of prostate-specific antigen in the plasma can indicate prostate cancer's existence.

C-reactive protein, often known as CRP, is a biomarker used to evaluate inflammation levels inside the body. Several inflammatory disorders, including rheumatoid arthritis, lupus, and cardiovascular ailments, have been linked to elevated CRP levels in patients' blood.

3. Prognostic Biomarkers

The third group comprises predictive biomarkers, which can predict the probability of a clinical event in individuals with the illness, such as the risk of disease recurrence or advancement. The following are some examples of predictive biomarkers:

Ki-67: This protein is a cell proliferation marker extensively employed as a predictive biomarker in breast, prostate, and other malignancies. Ki-67 has been shown to predict survival in patients with breast cancer accurately. There is a correlation between high levels of the protein Ki-67 and more aggressive cancers and worse outcomes.

BRAF is a gene often altered in malignancies other than melanoma, including lung and colon cancer. It is possible to anticipate the patient's response to targeted therapy by testing for BRAF mutations. BRAF inhibitors fall into this category. Patients with BRAF mutations may respond more to these medications and benefit from beginning treatment sooner than other patients.

4. Monitoring Biomarkers

The fourth category pertains to the monitoring of biomarkers, wherein the regular measurement of these indicators is conducted to assess the present condition of a disease or medical condition, as well as to quantify the level of exposure to a pharmaceutical product or an environmental pollutant. Tracking and evaluating biomarkers is an essential component of illness management and therapy.

The following are some examples of monitoring biomarkers:

Hemoglobin A1c, often known as HbA1c, is a biomarker that is used in the process of diagnosing and monitoring diabetes. The levels of HbA1c in the blood indicate the normal blood glucose levels over the last three months. These values may be used to monitor the course of the illness or the efficacy of therapies for diabetes.

Brain natriuretic peptide, often known as BNP, is a biomarker that monitors patients suffering from heart failure. BNP is secreted by the heart as a reaction to increasing pressure and volume, both characteristic of heart failure. Tracking levels of BNP may assist in determining the degree of heart failure and provide direction for treatment choices.

5. Predictive Biomarkers

The fifth category pertains to predictive biomarkers, which serve the purpose of identifying individuals who are more susceptible to experiencing either positive or negative effects as a result of their exposure to a medicinal product or environmental agent. These biomarkers have the potential to predict the result of an interaction between an individual and a medical product or environmental contaminant. The identification of suitable therapeutic interventions relies on the presence of predictive biomarkers. The HER2 protein serves as an illustrative instance of a predictive biomarker. This protein serves as an indicator for potential positive response to a certain targeted treatment in breast cancer patients.

The presence or absence of the **HER2/neu** protein in breast cancer HER2/neu is an overexpressed protein in some kinds of breast cancer. Predicting how well a patient will react to targeted therapy like trastuzumab (Herceptin) may be helped by testing for the HER2/neu status. Patients whose breast cancer tests positive for HER2/neu may benefit from starting therapy with trastuzumab early on since this may enhance their chances of survival.

The frequency of **EGFR** gene mutations in non-small cell lung cancer (NSCLC) EGFR is a gene usually changed in non-small cell lung cancer (NSCLC) cases. It is possible to estimate how well a patient will respond to targeted medicines by testing for the presence of EGFR mutations. These medications include gefitinib (Iressa) and erlotinib (Tarceva). Patients with EGFR mutations may respond more to these medications and benefit from beginning therapy sooner than other patients.

6. Response Biomarkers

The sixth group of biomarkers is known as pharmacodynamic/response biomarkers, and they are indicators that a biological reaction has been triggered in a person after they have been subjected to a medicinal product or an environmental contaminant. In clinical trials, these indicators are often used to evaluate the efficacy of novel medicines. Measuring the size of a tumor as a reaction to chemotherapy used in cancer treatment is an example of a pharmacodynamic and response biomarker.

These are some further examples:

LDL cholesterol levels may decrease as a result of using statins. Statins are a family of medications used to reduce cholesterol levels in people who suffer from high cholesterol. The decrease in LDL cholesterol levels (low-density lipoprotein cholesterol), which occurs directly from statin therapy, serves as the pharmacodynamic and response biomarker.

Blood pressure as a result of taking antihypertensive medication: Patients with hypertension often take medication to reduce their blood pressure while using antihypertensive medication. The decrease in blood pressure directly from therapy with these medications serves as the pharmacodynamic and response biomarker.

7. Safety Biomarkers

The final category pertains to safety biomarkers, which serve as indicators of the potential, presence, or degree of toxicity resulting from exposure to a medical product or environmental pollutant. This is the seventh and final category. Take, for instance:

Liver function tests, often known as LFTs, are a collection of blood tests that assess the amounts of enzymes and proteins generated by the liver. LFTs are also known as liver function assays. To monitor liver function and identify drug-induced liver damage (DILI), a possible side effect of certain drugs, liver function tests (LFTs) may be utilized as safety biomarkers.

The clearance of creatinine serves as an indicator of renal function and can be employed as a safety biomarker for the purpose of monitoring potential nephrotoxic effects of specific treatments, including chemotherapeutic drugs and antibiotics. Creatinine clearance is an amount of kidney function. Clearance of creatinine is a measure of kidney function.

Importance of Medical Tests

Tests in medicine are the backbone of today's healthcare system, and they play an essential part in diagnosing, monitoring, and preventing a wide variety of illnesses and diseases. These examinations are valuable resources that medical practitioners use to improve their understanding of the human body's complexities. As a result, they are more effective at diagnosing illnesses, determining the best course of treatment, and fostering general health and wellness. It is impossible to overestimate the significance of medical testing because of its role in the early identification, precise diagnosis, and efficient treatment of various health conditions.

The idea of early detection, an essential component that emphasizes the relevance of medical examinations, is the driving force behind this whole thing. During the early stages of many illnesses, the patients may or may not have any symptoms. This is true even for diseases that can potentially cause significant complications. The capacity of some medical examinations, such as blood screens and imaging scans, to identify abnormalities and deviations from normal physiological parameters may occur far before the manifestation of readily apparent symptoms. This early diagnosis allows medical professionals to respond quickly, beginning therapies that may arrest the course of illnesses or reduce their negative effects on an individual's health.

In addition, diagnostic tests play a significant role in ensuring correct diagnoses. When formulating complete assessments of their patient's health problems, medical professionals depend on various diagnostic tests and clinical examinations of their patients. By cross-referencing symptoms with test findings, medical professionals can confirm suspicions, exclude potential other diagnoses, and make educated judgments regarding the most effective treatment methods. In this way, medical tests improve the accuracy of diagnoses, lowering the likelihood of incorrect diagnoses and the accompanying possibility for patients to suffer damage.

The variety of medical testing goes all the way into the field of the treatment of chronic diseases. People who are living with chronic ailments such as diabetes, cardiovascular diseases, and autoimmune disorders need constant monitoring to evaluate the success of therapies and to avoid consequences. Blood tests should be performed frequently to monitor critical indications, which enables medical professionals to change treatment regimens as necessary. Patients are guaranteed individualized therapy thanks to this diagnostic testing and analysis cycle, which adapts to each patient's distinct physiological reactions and ever-evolving health requirements.

Medical tests excel in several areas, one of which is preventative healthcare, which exemplifies the old saying "prevention is better than cure." Even without symptoms, screening tests are intended to uncover risk factors or early signals of possible health problems. Screening tests are developed to identify risk factors or early signs of prospective health problems. Showing tests, such as mammograms, pap smears, and colonoscopies, are diagnostic procedures that may assist in early diagnosing breast, cervical, and colorectal cancers respectively. These tests allow people to take preventative measures to preserve their health, perhaps avoiding more intrusive treatments and attaining better results by recognizing anomalies before moving to advanced stages.

Medical testing covers various methodologies designed to shed light on a particular facet of an individual's health. Blood tests, for example, may provide insight into the body's inner workings by assessing blood composition, hormone levels, and the presence of biomarkers that are symptomatic of various illnesses. Radiological examinations, such as X-rays, CT scans, and MRIs, use modern imaging technologies to examine inside structures. This helps in the identification of fractures, cancers, and neurological problems. Examples of radiological tests include. Stress tests and pulmonary function tests are examples of functional testing. These tests examine how the body reacts to various stimuli, giving essential information about the cardiovascular and respiratory systems.

In addition to its monitoring and diagnostic functions, medical tests improve medical research and innovation. The data created by testing on a broad scale gives useful insights into the patterns of population health, the prevalence of illness, and the effects of therapy. Because of the quantity of information available, scientific discoveries are made, new medicines are developed, and public health policies that seek to improve the well-being of communities are informed. The enormous influence that medical testing, research, and advancement all have on the development of medical knowledge is highlighted by the interconnection between them.

PART 2:
THE ART OF LONGEVITY

CHAPTER 6:
MINDFULNESS AND MENTAL HEALTH

Stress and Its Effects on Longevity

The term "stress" may refer to any shift that burdens a person's physical, emotional, or mental health. Stress is your body's reaction to everything that needs attention or action.

Everyone goes through periods of stress to varying degrees. However, how you react to stressful situations significantly impacts your general health and well-being. Changing your environment may help manage stress, but it's not always the greatest solution. Altering your approach to react to a certain circumstance might be the most effective tactic at other times.

Signs of Stress

Stress can be short-term or long-term. Both can lead to various indications, but chronic tension can take a serious toll on the physique over a while and have ongoing health effects.

- Variations in mood
- Clammy or sweaty palms
- Decreased sex drive
- Diarrhea
- Difficulty sleeping
- Digestive problems
- Dizziness
- Feeling anxious
- Common sickness
- Grinding teeth
- Headaches
- Little energy
- Muscle tightness, particularly in the neck and shoulders
- Physical aches and pains
- Racing heartbeat
- Trembling

Identifying Stress

Recognizing Stress What does it feel like when you are stressed? What does it feel like to be under stress? It often adds to feelings of impatience, worry, overwork, and dissatisfaction in people's lives. You could feel physically exhausted, worn out, and unable to deal with the situation.

There are several methods to detect certain symptoms that you could be facing too much strain, including the fact that you might be stressed out. However, stress is not always simple to spot. There are instances when an evident cause brings on stress; however, there are occasions when even the seemingly little strains of everyday life, such as those brought on by job, school, family, and friends, may take their toll on your mind and body.

Keeping an eye out for the following signs may help you determine whether or not stress is affecting you:

- Behavioral symptoms such as difficulties focusing, worrying, anxiety, and forgetfulness, as well as psychological symptoms such as problems remembering things
- Manifestations of negative emotions include rage, irritation, irritability, or frustration.
- The naked eye may see signs, including a change in weight, an increase or decrease in menstrual cycle and libido, high blood pressure, and recurrent colds or infections.
- Behaviors such as not taking care of yourself, not having time to do the things you like, or depending on substances like alcohol or drugs to get through the day are indicators of a problem.

Effects on Longevity

Although stress is a normal and natural reaction to trying circumstances, it may harm our health and well-being if allowed to continue for an extended period.

According to several studies, stress may have a role in many health issues, including hypertension, cardiovascular disease, and even mortality at an earlier age. Stress may also harm our mental health, making us more susceptible to mood disorders such as anxiety, depression, and others.

The onset of chronic illnesses is one of the ways that stress might reduce our life expectancy since it plays a role in our development. A condition of persistent physiological arousal may result from chronic stress, and this state can cause harm to the body over time. This may have a role in developing infections such as cardiovascular illness, diabetes, and cancer, which can eventually result in mortality at an earlier age.

In addition, stress may harm our mental health, which can negatively affect our physical health and lifespan. Chronic stress may play a role in developing mood disorders such as depression and anxiety, both related to a range of adverse health significances, such as an amplified risk of cardiovascular disease and early mortality. Chronic stress can donate to the development of mood disorders such as depression and anxiety.

In addition, stress may result in the employment of unhealthy coping methods, such as excessive eating or drug addiction, which can further contribute to unfavorable health consequences.

In addition, stress may influence our actions and the choices we make about our lifestyle, which can substantially affect our health and lifespan. People under chronic stress may be more inclined to participate in habits that are detrimental to their health, such as smoking, drinking excessive amounts of alcohol, or eating an unhealthy diet. These habits are known to have a role in the development of chronic illnesses and have the potential to result in mortality at an earlier age.

It is essential to remember that not all forms of stress are the same and that certain stress conditions may be more detrimental than others. For instance, chronic stress brought on by social isolation or a lack of social support may be especially damaging. This is because social isolation has been connected to unfavorable health outcomes, including an increased chance of passing away earlier.

Not every person reacts the same way to stress, though; some people may be better able to shrug off the unfavorable consequences of stress than others. How an individual responds to stress may be affected by various factors, including their genes, personality, and the circumstances they've found themselves in throughout their lives.

Because it eases worry about future expenses, having an annuity might help someone live longer. Studies have indicated that persons who suffer financial stress are more likely to have inferior health outcomes, including a shorter lifespan, than those who do not experience financial stress. This may have a severe influence on both the physical and emotional health of an individual. An annuity, which guarantees a certain monthly income, may help alleviate money-related stress, which can benefit one's general health and may even lengthen one's life.

When coping with stress, having mental tranquility and a feeling of safety may be helpful. The assurance that one would continue to receive a certain amount of money each month might help one feel more secure and less anxious about the future. This may decrease stress levels and enhance mental health, positively influencing a person's lifespan.

A further benefit of annuities is that they may be structured to guarantee a steady income for the rest of a person's life, even if they live far longer than anticipated. People who are worried about outliving their funds or do not have any other potential sources of income during retirement may benefit tremendously from this option. An additional benefit of annuities is that they may provide a steady income unaffected by market changes.

However, a key point to remember is that annuities are not a one-size-fits-all solution and may not be appropriate for everyone. Both tension and the ability to relieve stress may benefit one's health; perhaps an annuity might be a part of the answer.

Mindfulness

Suppose you have your finger on the pulse of the health industry. In that case, you've likely heard of mindfulness exercises, which is a word that encompasses a variety of methods for bringing your attention to the moment that you're now in. You may have even experimented with various mindfulness meditations using the timer on your smartphone, an audio or video recording of a guided meditation, or an application on your mobile device. But let's face it: not everyone has the time (or the inclination) to carve out a certain period of the day for a dedicated meditation practice.

That's not a problem; the wonderful thing about practicing mindfulness is that you can incorporate it into even the most mundane aspects of your life. "some [people] have the misunderstanding that mindfulness means they requirement to sit cross-legged, eyes closed, and prepared to commit to at least 11 to 18 minutes." "Some [people] believe that mindfulness means they must sit cross-legged, eyes closed, and ready to commit to at least 11 to 18 minutes." However, this is unnecessary (unless that's your thing); you may still feel the advantages of mindfulness on your mental health by adopting straightforward strategies.

It is the practice of being present and aware, and it involves noticing whatever you are experiencing, perceiving, and thinking peacefully and without judgment. Mindfulness is a kind of meditation. This frame of mind may be employed in the here and now to help a person overcome difficult circumstances, such as being late to work or fighting with their spouse. Consistent practice may also generate long-term changes in how you interact with your ideas. She argues that doing this consistently over time may increase your capacity to deal with mental health challenges, namely anxiety, stress, and depression.

Knowing how to meditate is one type of mindfulness practice, but that doesn't mean it's the only method to become more aware of what's happening around you in the here and now.

But don't just take our word for it; we consulted several professionals to find fast and easy mindfulness exercises that can be incorporated into almost any routine. Suppose you're short on time or just searching for quick, easy stress relief. In that case, the following information will provide an overview of some of the advantages of practicing mindfulness and instructions on mindful awareness without meditation.

Mindfulness Exercises

1. Three-minute breathing space

This straightforward task can be accomplished within a three-minute timeframe, rendering it feasible even during periods of high workload. Mindfulness-based cognitive therapy, a therapeutic approach known for its efficacy in mitigating symptoms of stress, anxiety, and depression, frequently incorporates the utilization of this particular exercise.

The following explains how to put the "three-minute breathing space" into effect.

Put a three-minute countdown on the timer.

- Place yourself in a comfortable posture, preferably seated, although standing also helps, preferably in a somewhat quiet location (the restroom counts), and shut your eyes if you want. Take note of what is transpiring in your body and mind now. Do you take note of whatever you are encountering at this very moment?
- Focus all your attention on your breath and become aware of the feeling of air entering and leaving your body as you breathe in and out.
- Increase the scope of your zone of awareness to encompass your breathing and the rest of your body. Your posture, facial expression, or certain regions of muscular tightness may come to your attention. Again, pay attention to whatever sensations are occurring throughout your body.

2. Listening Mindfulness

One of her favorite methods to practice mindful living is concentrating on the noises around her. It requires focusing on a certain sound in your surroundings, which may be done anywhere, such as on a bus or in your kitchen. "Perhaps it's very obvious and audible, or perhaps it's something that's going on in the background," In all seriousness, everything goes.

After you have recognized a sound, such as far-off traffic, the constant hum of an air conditioner, or your neighbor's TV that is turned up too high, practice attentive listening with this simple method:

If you like the sensation, try closing your eyes. In such case, look about your area for a point you may gently glance at (relax your eyes and try not to concentrate on anything particular).

- Take a mindful listen to the sound. Pay attention to the note, the rhythm, and the loudness.
- Maintain as much coherence as possible with the sound. It is normal for your thoughts to stray sometimes; you only need to recognize this and return your attention to the sound. You may even try seeing your distracting ideas as being carried away from you on a balloon or carried down a stream by a leaf.
- When you feel like you've had enough, call it a day on the workout.

3. Mindful Eating

This requires paying attention to your food's flavor, appearance, and different textures. Try this out the next time you're enjoying a cup of coffee or tea, for example. You may pay attention to the temperature, the way the liquid feels on your tongue, and the degree of sweetness, or you could monitor the steam it puts off.

4. Mindful Moving, Walking or Running

Try to zero in on the sensation that your body is moving when you go out. When you go for a mindful stroll, you can notice the success of the air against your skin, the feeling of your feet or hands against the various textures on the ground or adjacent objects, and the many odors in the environment.

5. Body Scan

. In this practice section, you will carefully transfer your focus through the various regions of your body. You should begin at the very pinnacle of your head and work your way down to the tips of your toes. You could concentrate on the sensations of warmth, tension, tingling, or relaxation experienced in various places of your body.

6. Mindful Coloring and Drawing

. Instead of attempting to sketch a specific item, concentrate on the colors and the feeling of your pencil moving over the surface. You might use a coloring book designed for mindfulness or download pictures designed for coloring with mindfulness.

7. Mindful Meditation

Sitting still and concentrating on your breathing, thoughts, feelings in your body, or what you can perceive in your surroundings is required. If you find that your mind has wandered, you should bring it back to the here and now. Yoga, according to the experiences of many individuals, also makes it easier for them to concentrate on their breathing and pay attention to the here and now. Check out our article on the many forms of complementary and alternative treatments for further details on how meditation and yoga might help you.

Stress Log

Investigating Stressors:

Questions

1. What are the most prevalent stressors in your life right now?

Answer

2. Are there any repeating patterns or themes in your stressors?

Answer

3. Are there any stresses over which you have control or influence? Which ones are out of your hands?

Answer

4. What are the effects of your pressures on your physical health, emotional well-being, and general quality of life?

Answer

5. Are there any stressors that you think are unneeded or self-imposed? How would you go about reducing or eliminating them?

Answer

6. Are there any stressors that you find especially difficult or overwhelming? Why do they have such an impact on you?

Answer

Coping Mechanisms:

Question

7. What healthy coping methods do you now employ to deal with stress? How effective do you think they are?

Answer

8. Have you attempted any coping tactics in the past but found them unhelpful or harmful?

Answer

9. Do you have any favorite relaxation techniques or self-care activities for de-stressing? Describe how they help you.

Answer

10. Do you have any coping techniques that you'd like to develop or improve? What actions can you take to address them?

Answer

11. How do your coping techniques affect your interpersonal relationships? Are they concerned about your well-being?

Answer

12. Are there any coping methods that you've been meaning to use but haven't yet? What piques your interest in them?

Answer

CHAPTER 7:
QUALITY SLEEP AND RESTORATION

Importance of Sleep

There is no denying the significance of sleep as an integral component of our daily routines. However, because of the frantic and busy nature of our lives, we often give other things more importance before ultimately going to bed. Many of us watch hours upon hours of television and write emails when we really should be sleeping despite our fatigue.

Despite this, getting enough quality sleep is still one of the most essential things we can do for ourselves, and maintaining good sleep hygiene may lead to numerous advantages that you are probably not even aware of. Your ability to remember things and focus more sharply, as well as the strength of your immune system, lower blood pressure, and even help you lose weight, are all benefits of developing healthy sleeping habits.

However, there is also a strong connection between the amount of sleep you get and the state of your mental health. Getting enough sleep may help reduce the symptoms associated with stress, anxiety, and depression. This might imply less impatience unhappiness, and less of a sensation of being overwhelmed in daily living.

Getting enough sleep is quite important. The following information will assist you in achieving the highest quality of sleep possible.

Because of the "wear and tear" that our everyday activities do to our bodies, we need to give them time to relax and heal. According to a body of research, on average, those who get fewer than seven hours of sleep each day are at a greater risk of acquiring major medical conditions than those who get seven hours of sleep or more each night. Problems including diabetes, obesity, heart and blood vessel disease, stroke, and mood disorders like depression might fall into this category.

When we receive sufficient sleep, our brains are prepared to make choices, recall information, and respond promptly when required. People who have not had enough sleep struggle with their ability to concentrate, their memory, and other parts of thinking that need more complexity. These issues often become more severe when a person goes many days without getting enough sleep. People who are sleep-deprived often are unaware of the degree to which they are weary or how badly they perform at work or behind the wheel.

Recognize the specific sleep requirements of your body.

We have all been told that the optimal amount of sleep for a single night is eight hours. No two people have identical sleep requirements. You may get by just fine on six hours of sleep or need nine or more to feel totally refreshed. The key is to pay attention to your body and figure out what it requires from you by listening to it.

Establish a regular pattern of sleep.

Going from hitting the hay at 10 p.m. one night to pulling an all-nighter the next may generate long-term concerns for good sleeping habits. However, this may not be the case if your sleep patterns fluctuate greatly. (This is particularly relevant since our typical and established routines for the foreseeable future have been thrown off.) You may enhance the overall quality of sleep by keeping to a practice that requires you to go into bed and get out of bed at the same time each day.

Put down the phone and listen.

When it's getting near to sleep, using your phone, laptop, or tablet might be difficult for several reasons. You may feel more anxious if you spend time on social media; the same is true if you spend the latter portion of your evening feeling stressed over work emails.

However, the light emitted from your electronic device can also damage the excellence of your sleep. Phones and similar electronic devices emit a blue light that inhibits melatonin production in the brain. This hormone plays a role in modifiable sleep and circadian rhythms. This, in turn, results in poorer sleep quality for the user.

Stay away from both alcohol and coffee.

Caffeine and alcohol may negatively impact sleep and, as a general rule, should be avoided in the hours leading up to bedtime. This includes things like a cup of coffee or even a nightcap.

Because it is a stimulant, caffeine might keep you up for a long time after you had hoped to start dozing asleep. Meanwhile, drinking alcohol may disrupt your circadian rhythm and rapid eye movement (REM), a stage of the sleep cycle that benefits your health.

Try some caffeine-free herbal tea or, even better, just some water as an alternative to alcoholic beverages or espresso.

Don't simply lay there like that.

You keep rolling over and tossing your head. Despite your best efforts to force yourself to sleep and distract yourself with mindless activities like counting sheep, nothing seems to help. If you can connect to this predicament, then the following recommendation may come as a surprise to you.

If you're having trouble falling asleep, the best thing to do is to get up and try doing something else, like reading. This may seem counterintuitive, but it's been shown to be the most effective solution. This is done to prevent you from developing an unhealthy relationship between your bed and sleeplessness and to assist you in refocusing your attention on something else.

It's possible that you haven't given much thought to the correlation between getting enough quality sleep and maintaining a sound mental state. You may look forward to enjoying pleasant evenings and receiving the rest you need if you create beneficial habits and avoid activities and drugs that induce worry or arouse you.

Sleep Hygiene

Your sleeping patterns, which are directly related to the state of your health as a whole, are the focus of the field of sleep hygiene. The practice of daily routines that support your body's natural capacity to fall asleep, enter deep sleep, and remain asleep throughout the night is what we mean when we talk about having good sleep hygiene. Maintaining healthy sleeping habits increases the likelihood that you will awake feeling refreshed.

Your ability to fall asleep and continue asleep consistently may be improved by engaging in certain habits referred to as "sleep hygiene."

The following factors go into good sleep hygiene:

- What you put in your body, including the meals and drinks.
- Your routine for each day
- , the total amount of time spent being physically active during the day, and what you do in the evenings

Types of Sleep Hygiene

Generally speaking, one's degree of sleep hygiene may be categorized as excellent, bad, or fair. This indicates that you either have excellent habits, some good habits, and others that detract from a good night's sleep, or you have numerous bad sleep habits leading to poor sleep hygiene. If this is the case, you either have good habits or some good habits and others that detract from a good night's sleep.

The following characteristics represent what the Centers for Disease Control and Prevention considers to be a "good night's sleep" for the majority of adults:

- Achieving a sleep duration of seven hours or more every night
- After waking up, having a sense of having slept
- Having the sensation of being awake throughout the daylight hours indicates that one is not feeling rested.

It is considered bad sleep hygiene to receive less than the seven hours of sleep that are advised for each night. Lack of proper sleep hygiene may, over time, lead to sleep deprivation, which in turn increases the likelihood of developing sleep disorders such as insomnia. The Centers for Infection Control and Prevention states that more than one-third of all individuals in the United States are not getting enough sleep.

Inadequate sleep hygiene is recognized to be a risk factor for the following conditions as well:

- Overweight and obese
- Diabetes type 2 (T2D)
- Unhealthy levels of blood pressure
- Stroke and coronary artery disease
- Alterations in mood that are associated with mental health disorders

Changing how you normally sleep may help minimize the chance of developing a variety of health concerns, including those affecting your mental and physical health and sleep disorders.

The following are some of the recommendations made by specialists for enhancing your sleep hygiene:

- Create and maintain a sleep routine that you can adhere to daily, weekly, and even monthly.
- Ensure that the timetable you choose for your bedtime provides at least seven hours of sleep.
- Do not go into bed until you are completely prepared to sleep; for instance, do not head to bed sooner to browse through your phone's feed.
- Restrict usage of the bed to only sleeping and making love.
- Prepare your surroundings so that you have the best chance of succeeding (for example, a cold and dark room, comfortable bedding, etc.).

- Nicotine, coffee, and alcohol are stimulating drugs that should be limited or avoided entirely, particularly later in the day.
- Try not to stare at screens too close to when you need to sleep (for example, turn off all gadgets at least half an hour to an hour before bedtime).
- Restrict the quantity of food eaten and the kind of food ingested in the few hours leading up to bedtime (i.e., do not have a huge dinner (or one that is hot) or stuff yourself with heavy, processed food snacks immediately before attempting to fall asleep).
- Establish a relaxing ritual for the hour before you want to go to bed, such as taking a warm bath, washing your face, practicing meditation, or listening to a goodnight tale.
- Naps should not last more than 20 minutes and should be avoided if feasible.
- Engage in a sufficient number of physically active pursuits.

According to several pieces of research, maintaining appropriate sleeping hygiene is one of the most significant variables determining the quality of a person's sleep. To put it another way, making efforts to enhance your sleeping habits should always be considered a viable option. It has been established that getting a better night's rest may assist with more than simply sensations of restlessness. One research on college students, who are a high-risk population for sleep difficulties, showed that good sleep hygiene directly alleviated both depressive symptoms and feelings of general well-being. College students are a high-risk group for sleep disorders.

In addition to those discussed here, many more factors may contribute to a lack of quality sleep. Two factors include having a sleeping partner with poor sleep hygiene and experiencing chronic pain. Suppose you have trouble getting a better night's sleep after incorporating these suggestions into your normal routine. In that case, you may consider contacting your primary care physician and inquiring about the advantages of seeing a sleep expert or participating in a sleep study.

A person's sleeping routine is part of their "sleep hygiene." These habits that you engage in daily have a vast influence on the quantity and quality of sleep you receive, as well as the amount of time you can obtain each night. Not getting enough sleep (also known as having poor sleep hygiene) may, over time, lead to various health issues, including disorders affecting one's physical health and difficulties concerning one's mental health. You will be able to enjoy more soothing sleep and enhance your general health if you work on improving your sleep hygiene by following advice on how to get a better night's sleep.

Sleep log

Questions

1. On weekdays and weekends, what time do you usually go to bed?

Answer

2. On weekdays and weekends, what time do you generally get out of bed?

Answer

3. How much sleep do you hope to obtain each night?

Answer

4. Do you have a regular nighttime routine? If so, what exactly does it entail?

Answer

5. Are there any specific reasons or behaviors that routinely impair your sleep (e.g., coffee consumption, screen time before bed, stress)?

Answer

6. On a scale of 1 to 5, how would you estimate the quality of your sleep, with 1 being dreadful and 5 being outstanding?

Answer

7. How frequently do you have trouble getting asleep, remaining asleep, or waking up too early?

Answer

8. Do you have any reoccurring dreams or nightmares that keep you awake at night?

Answer

9. Do you have any sleep habits, such as tossing and turning, snoring, or sleepwalking?

Answer

10. Have you , such as an increase or reduction in sleep duration or a shift in your sleep-wake timetable?

Answer

Chapter 8:
Relationships and Community

Social Connection And Longevity

One of the most significant advantages of having meaningful social connections is their effect on one's physical health, which is essential to leading a long and happy life. Maintaining strong social relationships and a feeling of belonging may contribute to a longer lifetime, according to research that has repeatedly proven this to be the case. This is mostly the result of the following elements and effects.

Improved Health

People with strong social support networks have a lower risk of developing cardiovascular diseases, such as heart attacks and strokes. Social connection has been linked to improved immune system function and decreased levels of inflammation, which is associated with chronic diseases and accelerated aging.

Healthier Habits

People with strong social networks are more likely to adopt healthy routine choices, such as eating a balanced diet, going to the doctor for frequent checkups, and staying away from risky activities, such as smoking or drinking excessive alcohol. Having social ties may not only give the motivation and company needed to exercise regularly but can also contribute to improvements in one's physical fitness and general health.

Mental Exercise

Interacting with other people in various social circumstances is a great way to develop mental talent, creativity, and the ability to solve problems. Interactions with other people spark intellectual conversations, introducing us to fresh concepts, points of view, and information. This improves our cognitive function and extends our lifespan.

Emotional well-being

The alleviation of emotions of loneliness and isolation and the promotion of a sense of belonging and emotional well-being are outcomes of increased social interaction. Having a network of supportive contacts not only gives practical help during challenging times but also provides emotional support, which contributes to overall positive mental health and longevity.

It has been shown that having great social ties may favor adherence to medical treatments and therapies, leading to better management of chronic illnesses and improved overall health. After undergoing surgery, being diagnosed with a serious disease, or experiencing any other traumatic event, research has shown that people with strong social support networks tend to recover and heal far more quickly.

Meaningfulness and Life Satisfaction

The development of a feeling of belonging, purpose, and interconnection are all factors that contribute to an individual's level of happiness in life. Participating in social networks enables one to become part of a nurturing group that improves one's health in general and leads to the development of a life rich in purpose and satisfaction.

Relationships and Psychological Health

Not only is maintaining social connections crucial to our physical health, but it also has a significant impact on the mental health of each individual. By delivering various psychological advantages, including the following: Social interaction is one of the most important factors in enhancing mental well-being.

Calming Effects on Nerves and Stress

Social relationships provide a support network that helps reduce stress and anxiety by fostering greater levels of understanding and empathy. Successfully navigating difficult circumstances may benefit greatly from strong social relationships since they provide a feeling of safety and comfort.

Enhanced Sense of Pride and Assurance

Strong social ties may raise self-esteem and confidence by providing validation and acceptance from peers. Supportive relationships also provide opportunities for criticism and encouragement, which enables personal development and enhanced self-assurance.

Strengthened resistance

Strong social connections may be an invaluable asset for dealing with the difficulties of everyday life and gaining access to various opinions and potential solutions. Being a member of a social network also helps to cultivate a feeling of support and belonging, both of which contribute to increased resiliency and improved mental health.

Happiness and a better disposition

Participating in pleasurable social activities leads to the development of happy feelings and laughter, leading to a more comfortable and elevated state of mind resulting from engaging in activities and sharing experiences with others, generating a sense of happiness and connection.

Strategies for Enhancing Social Connection

The following tactics, which may help promote meaningful relationships and create a more rewarding and connected life, are geared toward those trying to strengthen their social ties.

Create new bonds

Leverage your connections by maintaining frequent contact with friends, family, and loved ones, participating in activities together, and creating experiences you can all enjoy together. Deeper relationships and stronger friendships may also be fostered and strengthened via talks through the use of active listening and the expression of empathy.

Build your social circle

The formation of new connections may be facilitated through activities in which participants engage as a group, such as joining a club or organization or volunteering for events or issues in the local community. Attending social meetings or events for networking gives possibilities to meet folks who have similar interests and widen one's social networks.

Accept and use modern technologies

Even when you are physically separated from friends and family, it is possible to keep in touch with them via various types of technology, such as social media platforms and other forms of the internet. Participating in online groups and forums devoted to topics that people have a common interest in may also assist you in meeting new people and expanding your network.

Conquer difficulties

Seek support from others or professional assistance if you have any social anxiety. Building confidence may be accomplished by taking baby steps outside your comfort zone, such as starting conversations or attending social events. The ability to effectively navigate social obstacles and develop new tactics may be greatly aided by participation in support groups or psychotherapy.

Create deep bonds with others around you

Stronger ties and a greater feeling of belonging may be cultivated by devoting one's time, energy, and attention to the cultivation of profound and significant relationships, as well as by expressing appreciation and thanks for the presence of others. Not only does the cultivation of meaningful relationships make our lives more fulfilling, but it also contributes to our general well-being, happiness, and longevity.

Building and Maintaining Healthy Relationships

The importance of relations in our lives cannot be overstated. They affect how content and healthy we feel. Building and maintaining any romantic, familial, friend, or work relationship requires time, energy, and conversation. This blog delves into the foundations of satisfying relationships and offers advice on improving yours.

Trust, respect, and open dialogue are the keystones for building strong relationships. Among the most important factors in fostering strong bonds are:

Good Listening Skills

Being a good listener is one of the most fundamental components of developing successful relationships, yet it's also one of the most underrated. The ability to maintain good relationships requires attentive listening. It demonstrates that you are interested in the other person's ideas and emotions, what they have to say, and that you appreciate what they have to say. The development of trust also relies heavily on effective communication. You may increase your comprehension of the other person's viewpoint and, as a result, your ability to make decisions and resolve conflicts as long as you actively listen to what they say. This helps cultivate mutual respect between the two parties in a relationship and can strengthen their connection with one another. Additionally, showing appreciation and thankfulness to the other person daily may assist in improving a relationship and maintaining its overall health.

Communication Skill

The ability to communicate effectively is essential to the development of strong connections. No matter the connection's nature (romantic, family, or platonic), it is critical to have effective communication skills and exhibit openness and honesty. Relationships are kept healthy, and difficulties are avoided during regular check-ins and dialogues. Participating in activities together is another way to develop connections and contributes to the upkeep of good relationships. Having great communication skills helps to create trust and understanding between people, which in turn leads to better relationships that are more enjoyable.

Empathy

Understanding the emotions of other people is the essence of empathy. It enables you to see things from their perspective and strengthens your connection with them. Demonstrating empathy may also increase communication, making settling problems simpler and locating areas of agreement. When you express empathy for another person, you communicate that you care about them and are prepared to listen to them and provide assistance. This contributes to creating a positive and supportive atmosphere, both of which are necessary for maintaining good relationships. Although developing empathy might be difficult at times, doing so can have a big positive effect on your connections with others.

Honesty and Trust

Building solid connections requires establishing and maintaining trust. When you are honest and reliable, you create a foundation of trust with the people closest to you, which paves the way for more candid and significant conversations between you and them. In addition, trust enables you to be vulnerable and real with the people you care about, which may lead to a deeper connection and a stronger relationship between you. In addition, having confidence in the other person gives you a sense of safety in the association. In a nutshell, trust is the foundation of any strong and meaningful connections with other people and the most important factor to consider while developing healthy relationships with others.

Maintaining Healthy Relationships

After you have established a strong connection with someone, it is essential to keep it alive. Maintaining good relationships needs both work and time and open and honest communication. Some important elements necessary for keeping healthy relationships include the following.

1. Regular Check-Ins

After you have established a strong connection with someone, it is essential to keep it alive. Maintaining good relationships needs both work and time and open and honest communication. Some important elements necessary for keeping healthy relationships include the following:

2. Time and Presence

For a relationship to flourish, both time and effort are required. In addition, it is essential to ensure that you make enough time to spend with the people who are important to you. Spending time with the people in your life exemplifies how committed you are to them, and this can be done in various ways, from going out to dinner to having a simple conversation. It demonstrates your desire to continue the relationship and respect for the people in your life. In addition, making an effort to spend time with the people you care about may help build a more profound feeling of love and support for one another.

3. Conflict Resolution

In any relationship, arguments and disagreements are inevitable. It is essential to deal with it in a healthy and courteous manner. Conflicts may be resolved, and good relationships are maintained by searching for solutions for both parties to reach an agreement. When disagreements are not fixed, they have the potential to become far more serious issues. When resolving problems and sustaining healthy relationships, excellent communication skills, empathy, and a willingness to compromise are essential. If necessary, it is not inappropriate to seek assistance from an impartial third party, such as a counselor or mediator. Keep in mind that resolving disagreements constructively will result in healthier relationships.

Cultivation and maintaining positive connections are essential to leading a meaningful life. It facilitates interpersonal relations, the formation of meaningful friendships, and the acquisition of a feeling of belonging in people. Relationships have the potential to provide us with support, love, and companionship, and they also play an important part in the maintenance of our general health and happiness. Whether it is a romantic connection, a relationship with a family member, a relationship with a friend, or a coworker, maintaining good relationships takes time, effort, and communication.

Social Health Log

Question

1. How would you rate the quality of your connections with family, friends, and strangers?

Answer

2. Do you have a support system in place on which you can rely on difficult times?

Answer

3. Do you have the ability to properly explain your thoughts and feelings to others?

Answer

4. Outside of work or school, how often do you engage in social activities and interactions?

Answer

5. Do you feel like you belong and are accepted in your social circles?

Answer

6. Are you stressed or unhappy because of any disagreements or unsolved difficulties in your relationships?

Answer

7. Are you willing to create boundaries in your relationships in order to safeguard your well-being?

Answer

8. How do you deal with peer pressure and make decisions that are consistent with your beliefs and objectives?

Answer

9. Are you actively attempting to broaden your social network and meet new individuals who share your interests?

Answer

CHAPTER 9:
PERSONAL ENVIRONMENT

The Importance of a Clean and Organized Space

Let's go into why having a clean and tidy room is like bringing a ray of sunshine into your life. Imagine this: you go into a room, and it's a clutter-free utopia. How does it make you feel? When everything is as it should be, you think you could take over the world. Now, picture the complete opposite, that there is disorder everywhere. Is it what you call a nice sight? There is more to it than meets the eye. Hold on to your hats because we're about to get down to the nitty-gritty of why maintaining order in your life may do wonders for your overall health and happiness.

Let's get the most important thing out of the way first: the mental game. A tidy environment is like a blank sheet of paper for your thinking. It's not hard to feel overwhelmed when you're surrounded by a sea of disarray all around you. Your ideas are as disorganized as the stack of paperwork now sitting on your desk. On the other hand, clearing out clutter and organizing may be analogous to pressing the mental equivalent of a reset button. You can concentrate more effectively, think more clearly, and even release your inner creative genius. It's like discovering a treasure map hidden in the chaos; suddenly, thoughts that had been buried spring to the surface.

And while we're on the subject of treasures, let's not overlook the time-saving magic of a well-organized home. Have you ever looked everywhere for your keys, only to discover them hiding behind a mountain of laundry? Yes, I've gone there and completed that. It's much easier to find things when the area is clean and organized. You won't have trouble finding what you want when you require it.

On top of that, think of all the priceless minutes you'll save by not having to go on a daily quest for things anymore. More time to spend on the activities that are important to you? That is undeniably a triumph!

However, this is not just about reducing the time you spend doing things; it may also improve your mood. The removal of clutter from your surroundings has the potential to improve your attitude significantly. As soon as you step into the room, the occupants give you a fist bump. You know that sensation when you've just finished cleaning up, and you can't help but let out a sigh of contentment? This is your spot letting you know, "Hey, I've got your back." When you're in a good mood, you are more inclined to face obstacles head-on and more likely to handle stress like a pro. It's like having a secret hideout where Superman goes to recuperate before going out to save the world.

Let's discuss the social scene now that we've gotten that out. Imagine bringing some guests to your apartment and having them walk into a paradise completely devoid of any mess. They report an immediate sense of calm and the impression that they have entered a warm and welcoming sanctuary. On the other hand, if your environment is disorganized, it will be difficult to conceal your constant feeling of humiliation. But have no fear! When you take the time to prepare your space, you increase the likelihood that you will host memorable gatherings and create cherished moments. Movie evenings, game nights, or anything else you may think of – the options are as limitless as the laughter that will be shared.

Now, let's confront the elephant in the room: cleaning up. We understand this is not the most thrilling item on your to-do list, and we apologize. However, constancy is the key to success in any endeavor. If you set aside a little time every day to clean up, you can avoid the mess that comes with it from becoming overwhelming. It is similar to doing routine maintenance to prevent the need for more extensive work. In addition, cleaning may even be turned into a therapeutic dance party by playing upbeat music or an exciting podcast in the background as you work.

In the great scheme of things, having a clean and organized room is not just about aesthetics but also about functionality. It's about making a haven for your thoughts, your time, your disposition, and the relationships in your life. It is about putting yourself in a position to be successful, welcoming each new day with a positive attitude, and appreciating the aesthetic value of a space devoid of clutter. Therefore, my friend, take that step, clean away the chaos, and watch as your life turns into a place where there is no limit to the possibilities available. Your body, brain, and heart will be grateful to you for doing so.

A long list of advantages comes with maintaining a tidy and organized house. Not only may it assist you in your personal life, but it may also make the process of selling your home or relocating your family to a location that is more suited to the needs of your group less difficult in the long term. Everyone will experience less stress during the day due to keeping things cleaned up and placed back where they belong. This alone will help folks who aren't feeling well to recover more quickly. If you keep at it, you'll be amazed at how much more time you have to appreciate your home instead of continuously seeking items already in the right place. Even though it could take some time to clear out all of the clutter from your house, if you keep at it, you'll be astonished at how much more time you have to enjoy your home.

Activity

1. An Attack Strategy

First and foremost, you must devise a strategy. Take a moment to plan before you start throwing stuff around. To stay on track, identify the areas that require the greatest cleaning, make precise targets, and develop a timeframe.

2. Storage Alternatives

Invest in storage solutions that are appropriate for your space. Having a specific area for your items, whether it's elegant baskets, shelves, or under-bed storage bins, is essential for keeping things organized.

3. Method of Three Boxes

This time-tested strategy is a lifesaver. Label three boxes or bags: 'Keep,' 'Donate/Sell,' and 'Trash.' Examine each object in the space and make rapid judgments on where it goes.

Be ruthless. When determining what to keep, consider if the object fulfills a function or provides you delight. If not, it may be time to say goodbye. Be tough when required but also emotional.

5. The Rule of One-In, One-Out

Adhere to the 'one-in, one-out' guideline to keep your area clutter-free. To keep things balanced, when you add a new item to your house, be prepared to say goodbye to something comparable.

6. Concentrate on one problem at a time

Don't overburden yourself by attempting to declutter your entire home at once. Concentrate on just one thing at a time, whether it's a room, a closet, or simply a drawer. This way, you'll be able to notice progress without feeling overwhelmed.

7. Time Administration

Set aside certain times for decluttering. It might be as little as an hour every day or as much as a weekend marathon. Maintain your commitment by sticking to your timetable.

8. Be Innovative in Your Organization

Keep things organized in imaginative and enjoyable ways. Mason jars for tiny objects, a shoe organizer on the back of doors, or a pegboard for tools may all make a big difference.

9. Digital Cleanup

Don't forget to clean your virtual life in this digital age. For a clutter-free computer experience, organize your emails, eliminate superfluous files, and clean up your digital gadgets.

10. Ongoing Maintenance

Decluttering is a continuous process. Make it a practice to perform brief decluttering sweeps on a regular basis to keep items from stacking up again.

CHAPTER 10:
INTEGRATING MIND AND BODY

Tai chi

Tai chi, a shortened form of the Chinese martial art tai chi chuan, is a mind-body exercise first developed in China. Tai chi has been practiced for millennia because of its many health advantages, 2including mental and spiritual well-being. In addition, the behavior is gaining more and more followers in the United States.

Tai chi is a low-impact workout that is becoming popular in modern times. Slow, soft motions characterize Tai chi. This ancient technique involves moving continuously while focusing on breathing and meditating. As you progress through a sequence of poses, you concentrate your attention on your body, as well as your thoughts and emotions. You take deep breaths.

When you practice tai chi, you should be standing in a comfortable squatting stance most of the time. Squatting at different depths allows you to tailor the challenge of the workout to your own needs. Alternatively, you might practice tai chi while sitting, which is an adaptation that makes the practice more approachable for those who have movement restrictions.

It is useful to study which type of tai chi is most suited to you if you are interested in pursuing tai chi to improve your health. The following are some broad characterizations of the five primary styles:

- Chen is the type of tai chi that has been around the longest and was developed in the 1600s. It combines quick, aggressive actions like leaping and hitting with slower, more delicate moves. Studies have shown that Chen-style Tai Chi may increase a person's balance and fitness level.
- Yang: Yang tai chi is characterized by its slow and steady movements, which combine wide stances with broad, sweeping motions. It is the tai chi style that is practiced the most often all around the globe. And it's possible that when you think about Tai Chi, this style springs to mind first. This is an excellent kind of tai chi for seniors since it is not difficult to learn.
- This well-known Wu style of Tai Chi was founded by Wu Quanyou, a student of the Yang family who taught Tai Chi. Wu is a calm and gentle kind of Tai Chi, much like

Yang. However, its more compact stance and forward-leaning attitudes may identify it from other horses.

- Sun Lutang, a scholar of Taoism and Confucianism, is credited with creating this relatively modern tai chi form. Because Sun Tai Chi involves more footwork than the other types, it may also be more beneficial for developing knee and ankle strength than the different kinds.

- The Hao method, also known as the Wu style at times, places an emphasis on qi, an internal life force often discussed in Chinese medicine. The movements of Hao Tai Chi are quite similar in appearance to those of other styles. However, the method places great emphasis on qi, and it is possible that only experienced Tai Chi practitioners should attempt to employ it.

Benefits

1. Improves both your balance and your mobility

Falls are the main cause of injury among people in this age range in the United States, affecting one in every four older individuals each year. According to several studies' findings, regular tai chi practice may help older people improve their flexibility and balance, lowering their chance of falling. The technique also allows persons with Parkinson's disease to combat reduced balance and movement, according to research.

The capacity of tai chi to strengthen proprioception may be responsible for these effects. Your ability to perceive the position and movement of your body is referred to as proprioception. Furthermore, it is essential for maintaining balance and moving about practically.

2. Develops strength in the lower body

You may not believe that exercises with minimum impact can boost the strength of your muscles. However, many studies demonstrate that practicing tai chi develops power in the lower body. One short research, for instance, investigated the impact of participating in a tai chi program on persons over 60. The research revealed that after 16 weeks of training, people who did tai chi had stronger knee flexors than those who did not.

3. Increases your self-assurance over your capabilities in the physical realm

The fear of falling is common among persons over the age of 65. It's possible that age-related changes like decreased muscle mass, worse eyesight, or other alterations are to blame for this worry. In addition, it may prevent individuals from engaging in physically active pursuits.

Tai chi has been shown to boost self-efficacy, which may be seen as a person's confidence in their capabilities. The possible gains in balance, strength, and mobility could explain this confidence increase. For example, one research discovered that older persons who practiced tai chi for eight weeks not only improved their credit but also experienced a reduction in their fear of falling.

Yoga

Pranayama, often known as yoga breathing, breathwork yoga, or simply pranayama, is a term that encompasses a variety of breathing exercises that may be performed on their own or as part of a yoga routine. Meditation is often practiced via the use of these various yoga breathing methods. The reduction of tension and anxiety and the improvement of breathing patterns are two other reasons why many people practice yoga breathing.

The breath is considered to be one's life energy while doing classical yoga or pranayama. Therefore, the significance of breathing in yoga lies in the fact that you may strengthen the connection between your mind and your body by deliberately engaging in the appropriate yoga breathing techniques. You may reach a level of mindfulness and open yourself up to a more complete awareness of the present by concentrating not only on your breathing but also on the yoga postures you are doing simultaneously.

Benefits of Yoga Breathing

- Reduces stress and anxiety: When you practice yoga breathing techniques for anxiety, you message your body's stress response that it is okay to relax and resume regular functioning. This allows you to feel less stressed and anxious.
- Doing these exercises before going to bed helps to relax both your body and mind, enabling you to enter a more peaceful state and remain asleep for longer.
- Using these techniques may help you establish a level of peace throughout your body and mind, much like performing yoga breathing exercises to reduce stress can help to calm the body.
- Yogic breathing may assist in maintaining an appropriate blood pressure level, which is particularly beneficial for those prone to surges in blood pressure while under stress. This effect has the additional benefit of lowering blood pressure.
- One of the most significant advantages of practicing yoga with a diaphragmatic breathing pattern is improving a person's respiratory health. This is accomplished by strengthening the muscles of respiration and enhancing the body's airways.
- Enhances cognitive functions, such as memory and concentration. Improving your breathing via yogic breathing exercises may help you improve your cognitive functions, such as your memory and concentration.

- Those trying to beat their addictions may utilize yogic breathing to lower the intensity of their cravings and quiet their racing thoughts. This assists in the management of addiction.
- The higher oxygen levels and carbon dioxide tolerance that occur inside your body due to practicing yogic breathing may significantly contribute to your increased energy levels and ability to perform well in physical activities.
- Yoga breathing not only helps you breathe more correctly, but it also helps you better filter the air around you, which ultimately increases your body's resistance to illness.
- Yogic breathing may be utilized at times of high stress to assist in calming and relaxing the body and mind. This can be helpful in the management of symptoms of post-traumatic stress disorder (PTSD). This may make it easier for clinicians to manage the symptoms of post-traumatic stress disorder (PTSD).

Spiritual Practices and Their Role in Longevity

The eternal search for ways to live a long and healthy life. Since the beginning of time, we have been on this quest. We have been looking for elixirs of youth that would last forever, we have been participating in scientific research, and we have been reading medical publications. But what do you think? Finding one's spiritual center may sometimes be a deceptively easy step toward a long and fruitful life. But it can also be one of the most important. You did indeed hear it correctly. Spiritual practices, which all too frequently get shoved to the side during our busy lives, may play a critical part in determining how many candles you can blow out on your birthday cake.

To begin, let's speak about how stressful things may be. It is deadly in every sense of the word. Problems with the heart, excessive blood pressure, and everything else you can think of. The unpleasant party visitor who overstays their welcome and leaves your home in a disorganized state is analogous to the stress that people experience. However, here's the kicker: spiritual practices such as meditation and mindfulness are like those in charge of cleaning up. They go in, assist in resetting, and suddenly, your mental home is back in order. You're doing more than simply giving your mind a vacation when you frequently tune into your inner world; you're strengthening your body's natural defenses against illness. Studies have indicated that persons who meditate or pray regularly have lower amounts of the stress hormone cortisol in their bodies. If you were wondering, that hormone is produced in response to stress. A lower cortisol level correlates with a happy heart and a longer life.

Okay, let's move on to the next topic, the community component. Are you familiar with the proverb, "It takes a community?" In any case, it's not only for raising children but also for becoming older. Many forms of religious and spiritual practice are conducted in groups, such as attending religious services, visiting temples, or participating in meditation retreats. Believe me when I say that the community is important. Research printed in the Journal Medicine found that good social interactions increase your chances of living by fifty percent. Just give it some thought. You are not just reciting prayers or chanting mantras; you are strengthening your social safety net and, thus, increasing your life expectancy. It's almost like getting something for nothing!

But hold on, there's more to it. Have you ever heard of the term telomeres? These are the little caps at the end of the strands of DNA in your cells that prevent them from unraveling. They are similar to the plastic tips that are found on shoelaces. The length of these men and their effectiveness decreases as we age. However, do you have any guesses about what may be of assistance? You probably guessed correctly: various spiritual activities. People who meditate regularly have telomeres that are much longer. When telomeres are longer, cell function is improved; when cell function is improved, a person lives a longer and healthier life. Sitting motionless and concentrating on your breath is almost as though your cells are receiving a maintenance checkup. That is very awesome to hear.

Okay, but let's not lose sight of the bigger issue here. Developing one's spiritual practice may infuse one's life with meaning and purpose. Have you ever had the experience of feeling like you're simply going through the motions, as if you're just locked in a dull cycle of eating, sleeping, working, and repeating? This is where a spiritual perspective might be helpful. It acts as a navigation system for your spirit, pointing you toward a life with deeper significance. You can get a sense of perspective when you establish a connection with something bigger than yourself; this might be God, the universe, or even simply the splendor of nature. The difficulties appear more manageable, the good times seem more abundant, and the length of life seems to increase.

Also, spirituality's positive impact on one's mental health should not be ignored. Anxiety, sadness, and the whole shebang are not simply conditions that affect the mind; they are also elements that may shorten the amount of time you have left in this world. Spirituality, please meet mental health and mental health, please meet spirituality. They greet one another with a handshake, and after some small talk, an alliance that will hopefully last a long time is formed. Attending religious services consistently was connected with a decreased risk of suicide, according to research published in the journal JAMA Psychiatry. Even if you don't have serious problems with your mental health, engaging in spiritual activities may provide you with a feeling of calm and mental clarity that can help protect you from the negative effects of the stresses of everyday life. It's almost like having a Zen-based emotional shield around your body.

And while we're at it, here's something to mull about. The spiritual path fosters admirable characteristics such as compassion, forgiveness, and thankfulness. Have you ever nursed a grudge? It's not enjoyable, and it's physically bad for your heart. Yeah, that about sums it up. Remember that carrying around wrath and resentment is a source of stress? And stress is the unwelcome visitor to the party we discussed previously.

Conversely, forgiving someone is like showing stress on the door and then shutting it. Not only will you see an improvement in your mental health via the cultivation of compassion and forgiveness, but you'll also be doing your body a huge favor. It's like getting two things done at once, or, to put it another way, like saving two people's lives with one act of kindness.

Activity

1. **Goals:** First and foremost, choose what you want to accomplish with your program. Do you wish to lower your stress, increase your flexibility, or enhance your mood?
2. **Mindfulness Practices:** Being present in the moment is central to mindfulness. To assist you concentrate your thoughts, you can use meditation, deep breathing techniques, or even progressive muscle relaxation.
3. **Choose physical activities that you enjoy**. Yoga, tai chi, or even a simple daily stroll will help you move your body while keeping you balanced.
4. **Choose a time that works for you**. Consistency is essential, whether it's in the morning to jumpstart your day or in the evening to unwind.
5. **Create a dedicated area for your routine**. It might be a quiet area of your home or a neighboring park. Having a designated area might help you stay to your habit.
6. **Equipment:** Depending on the activities you choose, you may require certain equipment. A yoga mat is useful for practicing yoga. Tai chi may need the use of suitable apparel and footwear.
7. **Consider seeking advice if you are new to mindfulness or particular activities**. To guarantee that you're doing things correctly, you may take classes or use online tutorials.
8. **Change things up**! Incorporate new workouts or mindfulness methods to keep your practice interesting. This keeps you interested and minimizes boredom.
9. **Music:** Relaxing music might enhance your experience. To accompany your regimen, make a playlist of your favorite peaceful tracks.
10. **Share your adventure with friends or family for moral support.** Having a support system might assist you in remaining motivated and accountable.

11. **Patience:** Rome was not built in a day, and a flawless mind-body habit is not either. Be kind to yourself, and don't get frustrated if you skip a day or encounter difficulties along the road.

12. **Adaptability**: Life may be unpredictably unexpected. Prepare to alter your routine to changing situations. If you are unable to complete your typical regimen one day, locate a shorter alternative.

13. **Reflection:** Take time to consider how your habit affects your life. Are you feeling better at ease? Has your adaptability increased? Based on your observations, modify your regimen as appropriate.

14. **Finally, yet importantly,** have some fun! Your mind-body regimen should make you happy and calm. If you are not having fun, do not be scared to change things around.

CONCLUSION

It is necessary to reflect on our trip through the complicated path of aging biology, genetics, nutrition, and mental well-being as we turn the last page of "Outlive Workbook". We have delved deeply into the scientific study that explains the natural process of aging and investigated the nuanced art of nourishing our physical, emotional, and mental capabilities. What is the overarching goal? To live longer, healthier lives that are filled with meaning, pleasure, and energy in addition to increased longevity.

Because of the uncertainty that is inherent to life, there are no assurances. However, what this workbook provides is empowerment in the form of a set of skills and information that will help you to guide the trajectory of your life toward maximum longevity. Your participation in the quizzes, self-evaluations, and activities has not only given you a momentary look into the science of longevity but it has also helped shape a tailored strategy that resonates with your life circumstances and ambitions.

Keep in mind that the objective of pursuing longevity is not just to add more years to one's life, but rather to add more life to one's years. It's about making the most of your time, making meaningful relationships with other people, taking care of your body, stretching your intellect, and cultivating an unending improvement and development attitude.

Let this workbook be a continuous companion for you as you continue on your path as you go ahead. You should repeat the exercises, keep your plan up to date in light of the changes that life brings, and keep in mind the great potential that lies within you to mold the future of your health and longevity.

We are grateful that you have chosen to make "Outlive Workbook" a part of the journey that is your life. Let us toast not just the number of years ahead of us but also the quality of those years. I want you on your path to be blessed with enlightenment, good health, and an unending enthusiasm for life.

Made in the USA
Columbia, SC
15 October 2023

24486892R00050